Hacking Healthcare

Fred Trotter and David Uhlman

Beijing · Cambridge · Farnham · Köln · Sebastopol · Tokyo

Hacking Healthcare
by Fred Trotter and David Uhlman

Copyright © 2013 Fred Trotter and David Uhlman. All rights reserved.
Printed in the United States of America.

Published by O'Reilly Media, Inc., 1005 Gravenstein Highway North, Sebastopol, CA 95472.

O'Reilly books may be purchased for educational, business, or sales promotional use. Online editions
are also available for most titles (*http://my.safaribooksonline.com*). For more information, contact our
corporate/institutional sales department: (800) 998-9938 or *corporate@oreilly.com*.

Editor: Andy Oram	**Cover Designer:** Karen Montgomery
Production Editor: Jasmine Perez	**Interior Designer:** David Futato
Copyeditor: Teresa Horton	**Illustrator:** Robert Romano
Proofreader: O'Reilly Production Services	

Revision History for the First Edition:
    2011-10-07   First release
    2012-10-08   Second release
See *http://oreilly.com/catalog/errata.csp?isbn=9781449305024* for release details.

ISBN: 978-1-449-30502-4

[LSI]

1349704147

Table of Contents

Preface

Thousands of computer experts seek to enter the field of healthcare information technology (health IT or HIT), and they are needed. In December 2009, the U.S. Department of Health and Human Services estimated that computerization just within the healthcare industry will add a need for 50,000 new IT staff.[1] These recruits to healthcare will bring valuable lessons learned through work in online commerce sites, financial institutions, or large corporate and university campuses, but they will be fundamentally bewildered during their first year or so at a hospital or clinic.

Meaningful use is the focus of this book because it is the term used in the Health Care Reform and Health IT Stimulus Act (HITECH, part of the American Recovery and Reinvestment Act of 2009) to encompass a vision of improved healthcare through computerization and digital networks. There's a great deal of nervousness among U.S. healthcare providers about meaningful use. Can they push their organizations into the twenty-first century vision it represents? Will their IT systems really support it, and even if certified for meaningful use this year, will the systems support it in the future? And even if hospitals and clinics adhere to the letter of the law, will they really reap the benefits promised by health IT?

So meaningful use, for us, stands for much more than a set of requirements in a particular set of U.S. regulations. It represents a form of care that empowers the patient, that does not harm her, that promotes long-term health, and that is affordable for everyone. To realize this vision, IT staff in hospitals and clinics have to understand how their particular institutions work and what roles they play.

This book, so far as we know, is the first candid attempt to bridge the gap between clinicians and IT staff. It explains the factors that make healthcare settings different from other jobs and academic settings that computer staff may have come from—and that make the healthcare settings different from each other—so that readers enter these settings with a deep respect for their practices. We will not be reticent about sources

---

1. Help Wanted: Skilled Health IT Workforce to Modernize Health Care A Message from Dr. David Blumenthal, National Coordinator for Health Information Technology (*http://healthit.hhs.gov/portal/server.pt/community/healthit_hhs_gov__university_training__facts_at_a_glance/1430*), December 24, 2009.

of resistance to new computing opportunities. But we will give you a starting language for discussing the path to and beyond meaningful use.

We don't delve too deeply into technical details here, because they are fast changing. If we explained how to set up S/MIME for a direct email gateway, you might find that better options already exist when you get into the workplace. If we explained how to interact with the fields of a CCD, you would probably find that these fields are undergoing constant change and that much of the data you deal with requires a different format. So this is a different type of technical book: a book that gives you a context for choosing and implementing the right technology for your organization.

Audience

We've directed our writing mostly at computer professionals, but this book can still be valuable for doctors, other clinicians, and other staff at healthcare institutions as well. We occasionally use terms from computer science and programming that will be familiar to people from those fields and might not be known to other readers. But we think that even the general reader can skip over technical details that he or she doesn't understand, and learn a lot about how to talk to other people about computers and networking in healthcare.

Organization

The chapters in this book are as follows.

Chapter 1, Introduction
> An overview of the topics of this book, a discussion of differences between medical settings, and an overview of meaningful use, which will be fleshed out later in the book

Chapter 2, An Anatomy of Medical Practice
> The wide variety of ways healthcare settings deal with patients and staff, and how workflows vary

Chapter 3, Medical Billing
> A candid investigation into how providers charge for care and how they get paid

Chapter 4, The Bandwidth of Paper
> An explanation of how deeply embedded paper records are in U.S. clinical settings, and what you need to do to migrate to electronic records

Chapter 5, Herding Cats: Healthcare Management and Business Office Operations
> A review of what happens just outside the doors of the treatment room where administrative and IT staff perform traditional business operations

Chapter 6, Patient-Facing Software
> A detailed look at how patients can use technology to become participants in their own care, including such notions as personal health records, online communities, and the quantified self

Chapter 7, Human Error
> A discussion of the most pressing problem in healthcare: avoidable errors, and how electronic records can both help and exacerbate the problems

Chapter 8, Meaningful Use Overview
> A concise breakdown of the requirements for becoming meaningful use compliant

Chapter 9, A Selective History of EHR Technology
> It is not possible to cover every important event in the history of a technology, but this discusses some of the highlights.

Chapter 10, Ontologies
> Vocabularies, jargon, classification systems for diseases and treatments, and other elements of making sense of information

Chapter 11, Interoperability
> A review of the technologies to exchange electronic healthcare records and the processes and systems that enable the process

Chapter 12, HIPAA: The Far-Reaching Healthcare Regulation
> When is health data covered under HIPAA, and what does that mean for your technology deployments?

Chapter 13, Open Source Systems
> Several comprehensive and fully featured systems exist to permit meaningful use compliance while using only open source software; these offerings provide an important reference and public resource for understanding meaningful use in technological terms or for real-world use

Appendix, Meaningful Use Implementation Assessment
> A checklist to help you determine how close your institution is to becoming meaningful use compliant

Conventions Used in This Book

The following typographical conventions are used in this book:

Italic
> Indicates new terms and emphasis.

 This icon indicates a warning or caution.

Using Code Examples

This book is here to help you get your job done. In general, you may use the code in this book in your programs and documentation. You do not need to contact us for permission unless you're reproducing a significant portion of the code. For example, writing a program that uses several chunks of code from this book does not require permission. Selling or distributing a CD-ROM of examples from O'Reilly books does require permission. Answering a question by citing this book and quoting example code does not require permission. Incorporating a significant amount of example code from this book into your product's documentation does require permission.

We appreciate, but do not require, attribution. An attribution usually includes the title, author, publisher, and ISBN. For example: "*Hacking Healthcare* by Fred Trotter and David Uhlman (O'Reilly). Copyright 2013 Fred Trotter and David Uhlman, 9781449305024."

If you feel your use of code examples falls outside fair use or the permission given above, feel free to contact us at *permissions@oreilly.com*.

Safari® Books Online

Safari Books Online is an on-demand digital library that lets you easily search over 7,500 technology and creative reference books and videos to find the answers you need quickly.

With a subscription, you can read any page and watch any video from our library online. Read books on your cell phone and mobile devices. Access new titles before they are available for print, and get exclusive access to manuscripts in development and post feedback for the authors. Copy and paste code samples, organize your favorites, download chapters, bookmark key sections, create notes, print out pages, and benefit from tons of other time-saving features.

O'Reilly Media has uploaded this book to the Safari Books Online service. To have full digital access to this book and others on similar topics from O'Reilly and other publishers, sign up for free at *http://my.safaribooksonline.com*.

How to Contact Us

Please address comments and questions concerning this book to the publisher:

O'Reilly Media, Inc.
1005 Gravenstein Highway North
Sebastopol, CA 95472
800-998-9938 (in the United States or Canada)
707-829-0515 (international or local)
707-829-0104 (fax)

We have a web page for this book, where we list errata, examples, and any additional information. You can access this page at:

   http://www.oreilly.com/catalog/9781449305024

To comment or ask technical questions about this book, send email to:

   bookquestions@oreilly.com

For more information about our books, courses, conferences, and news, see our website at *http://www.oreilly.com.*

Find us on Facebook: *http://facebook.com/oreilly*

Follow us on Twitter: *http://twitter.com/oreillymedia*

Watch us on YouTube: *http://www.youtube.com/oreillymedia*

Acknowledgments

Our deep thanks go to the myriad reviewers, commenters, and critics who have served to help improve this text. Health IT is an expansive subject and it is very easy to get the details wrong. Special thanks goes to Dave deBronkart (e-patient Dave), Shahid Shah, Will Ross, Alesha Adamson, Jacob Reider, Vincent Fitts, and Chris Bacon for reading the text online and providing detailed comments. Gary Teichrow, Mike Hogarth, and Peter Hendler provided specific technical guidance on various issues. Andy Oram, our O'Reilly editor, did an amazing job of both editing and effective task management.

CHAPTER 1

Introduction

Advances in the delivery of healthcare have allowed Americans to live longer, healthier lives than ever before, but costs are out of control and medical errors are dangerously common. Such is the universal assessment of healthcare in the United States and it is widely acknowledged that healthcare information technology (health IT or HIT) can help. What's largely missing from the literature in the healthcare field is precise and actionable advice to IT staff and the clinicians who work with them to make the health IT transformation a reality. This book was written to start filling the void.

About the same number of people die each year from medical errors as from automobile accidents. Heart disease and cancer kill the most people in the United States, more than 500,000 each year. But stroke and lung diseases are each responsible for about 100,000 deaths each year—and scandalously, so are medical errors. Medical errors are notoriously difficult to track, given our litigious society, so we really do not know how many deaths that statisticians attribute to cancer or heart disease were also related to medical errors. But given the high likelihood that errors are implicated in some of these deaths, it is possible that medical errors could be the third leading cause of death in the United States.

In 2000, the release of a report titled "To Err is Human" by The National Academies (the country's leading research institute in medicine) highlighted the astonishing rate of medical errors. It was a wake-up call to the healthcare industry, but the problem is still little known among the public, and in the absence of organizational change and technical adoption, little has been done to fix the problem.

Cost now dominates the news about healthcare. Some estimates put healthcare in the United States at one sixth of the total national economy. Healthcare insurance costs that go up sometimes 15% or 20% a year are threatening to bankrupt many local governments and forcing them to cut back services in a poor economy. Other wealthy nations spend much less on healthcare, but still have similar or better levels of healthcare quality.

HIT, or more colloquially "software for clinicians," promises to address these two fundamental problems: to lower healthcare costs and improve patient safety.

The Veterans Affairs (VA) hospitals in the United States offer the most substantial example of systemic improvements in quality using health IT. Since the 1970s, the VA has gone from a system with a reputation as a low-quality provider to a system widely regarded as the safest and most effective healthcare delivery system in the world. VA hospitals almost obsessively measure the quality of the healthcare they deliver, and they have the numbers to back up the assertion that they are tops. The quality of the VA system, and its focus on health IT to deliver quality, is documented in the book *The Best Care Anywhere* by Phillip Longman. Rather than quote all of the quality statistics in that and many other books, we will relate two simple cases that show the power of leveraged health IT systems at the VA.

In 2004, the drug company Merck voluntarily withdrew Vioxx from the market. Vioxx had been used to treat chronic pain, but it had become clear, over time, that Vioxx had a dangerous side effect: fatal heart attacks. Evidence also emerged that by 2000, Merck had evidence that Vioxx was dangerous. The fact that Vioxx was approved by the Food and Drug Administration (FDA), and that it was used so long after it was known to be dangerous, has been the subject of intense scrutiny.[1]

But years before the healthcare profession as a whole was aware of the dangers of Vioxx, the VA discovered on its own that it was a dangerous medication. Data from the VA's electronic healthcare record, VistA, had alerted the VA that something was amiss with Vioxx. The VA took steps to ensure that Vioxx was prescribed only with careful monitoring and only in special circumstances, a drug of last resort. By doing so, the VA saved thousands of lives.

The second case is the level of integration experienced by VA hospitals. If a veteran receives treatment in one VA hospital for a decade and then moves to another hospital, even another state, he can expect a decade's worth of VA records to be available at the new hospital on his first visit. The VA has achieved near-complete health data liquidity for its covered veterans. In comparison, most other healthcare systems typically still use fax machines to exchange health information.

This is the stage that has been set for health IT. Medical errors are too common, costs are out of control, and effective deployment of computerized records and workflow can dramatically reduce these errors and lower costs. This book will discuss preventable medical errors in detail, and show how many different health IT functions, from health data exchange to different types of reporting, can help to address healthcare quality and reduce medical errors.

---

1. Vioxx, the implosion of Merck, and aftershocks at the FDA (*http://www.thelancet.com/journals/lancet/article/PIIS0140-6736%2804%2917523-5/fulltext*)

Health IT and Medical Science

Most of those who are deeply involved in healthcare IT have chosen this field as a mission or vocation, rather than merely a career. Many health IT professionals have historically taken substantial pay cuts compared with IT professionals in other areas (although this is improving now). Many of us work in this industry because we lost a loved one to a simple medical error, or some other failure of the healthcare delivery system. For many of us, this is our life's passion. To us, "reducing the costs and improving the quality of healthcare" is a dry and frail description of our ambition for health IT. To paraphrase Steve Jobs, we want to make a dent in the human condition.

Before we can talk about what that next stage will be like, we should acknowledge that it will not be anything like past medical advances. Pasteur's microorganism model of disease, Darwin's theory of evolution, Florence Nightingale's redefinition of nursing, Roentgen's X-ray, or perhaps even the discovery of DNA by Watson and Crick are examples of game-changing insights. These are classic examples of massive improvements in healthcare delivery that come from a new fundamental insight. The improvements to healthcare that happen because of computerization will not be a revolution, but an evolution.

Fundamental to the ambitions in the health IT community is a humble acknowledgment that these huge game-changing insights are rare. We can expect fewer and fewer of them as the science of medicine progresses. Instead, medicine must now begin the difficult work of chronicling the immense complexity of a single cell's DNA, proteins and other structures, and how that cell cooperates with other cells in the human organism. We can no longer expect that individual insights will leap medical science forward, but instead the medical community will make hundreds of thousands of small incremental advances on tens of thousands of diseases.

If we hope to continue the rate of improvement in healthcare we must find a way to coordinate the contributions of countless clinicians, researchers, and patients. To make any sense out of the genotype, we must have a understanding of phenotype —the manifest characteristics of individuals, such as their age, weight, medical symptoms, mental status, and many other measurable traits —than is several orders of magnitude deeper than it is today. We must be able to gather and parse a hundred times more data about each patient than we do today, and we must be able to compare that rich data among millions of patients. Today, the sciences and the software that support clinical trials, genomics, and standard clinical operations are separate and distinct, with infrequent overlap. Tomorrow, these disciplines will merge into a single enormous effort to improve healthcare. Science on this scale is impossible without mass high-quality computerization. There is no reason why all of this cannot be accomplished while respecting patient privacy and other basic notions of human dignity.

We hope to use technology to improve every aspect of healthcare. We hope to create information systems that help to turn medicine into a higher art and a higher science.

As you can imagine, with such ambitions, the health IT community frequently has delusions of grandeur. But we also suffer from frequent and stifling disillusionment. Although most of us agree that health IT has tremendous potential, progress in the field has been far too slow. We have a few good examples, like the VA with VistA, demonstrating that massive improvements to healthcare delivery are possible by leveraging technology. But we must admit that although we have a few good examples, we have countless examples of failure.

The authors of this book believe both that health IT has tremendous potential and that health IT is surprisingly difficult. As we discuss its difficulties, and the methods that have been used to successfully overcome them, we hope to avoid the pessimism that is all too common in health IT. Having said that, when pessimism and discouraging voices abound, it is often for good reason. There are real pitfalls in health IT, and this book should show you how to avoid many of them.

Meaningful Use and What It Means to Be an EHR

Health IT has changed tremendously over the last few years. The biggest change in the United States has come from the simple phrase "meaningful use." The term is now solidly entrenched as the catchphrase for health IT in the United States. Most important, meaningful use represents reasonable first steps toward the long-term potential for health IT. For better or worse, the dreams and ambitions of the healthcare informatics industry are tied to the concept.

The phrase first appeared in the Health Information Technology for Economic and Clinical Health (HITECH) portion of the American Recovery and Reinvestment Act of 2009 (ARRA). ARRA defined that a substantial portion ($20 billion) of the money set aside by Congress to stimulate the United States economy after the financial and foreclosure crisis would go to doctors and hospitals who "meaningfully use" clinical software. The HITECH act was the first step in President Barack Obama's comprehensive plan for healthcare reform. Clinicians would receive the stimulus money to pay for software to improve the delivery of patient care.

The bill referred to that software by the currently popular term *electronic health record* (EHR) software. But software designed to improve the delivery of clinical care has been around for decades, under different names. Such software has been called computerized patient records (CPR), electronic medical records (EMR), electronic health records (EHR), and countless other similar names with corresponding abbreviations. Even more confusing, there was no set definition of what this class of software was supposed to achieve. Unlike software products such as word processors, spreadsheets, or database storage engines, which all have well-understood definitions, the software category of EHR has meant very different things to different people. Passionate users would assume that EHR software meant the features that they wanted. Developers assumed that EHR meant the set of features in the software that they had developed. Of course, different users and different developers rarely agreed on which features were the most important. Dr. Ignacio Valdes (a medical doctor possessing a master's degree in computer science with a stellar reputation in the health IT community) has frequently said, "For decades, doctors had no idea what they wanted, and software developers have given it to them."

For clinicians, these terms served as a source of confusion and frustration. It was totally unclear what different names implied about the functionality of the software. Even a few years ago, when a doctor would say "I want an EHR!", the right response from a health IT software vendor would have been "Fine, exactly what do you mean by EHR?"

The meaningful use EHR certification requirements have finally dictated exactly what EHR software needs to do for the doctors, hospitals, and other eligible providers who purchase, use, and deploy the software to receive payments from the ARRA-HITECH stimulus plan. In fact this has made the meaningful use requirements even more important than the term EHR. What is an EHR? That which can be used by a clinician to achieve meaningful use.

Why So Late?

IT experts, as well as the general public, often fail to ask one simple question that will help focus any discussion of healthcare informatics: *Why did the United States healthcare industry need to be paid to computerize?* Every other industry computerized when, and to the degree that, computerization held intrinsic competitive advantages for members of that industry. Market forces compelled computerization, and companies that refused or resisted the move to computerization were squeezed out by competitors who were leaner and faster as the result of automated processes.

This has not happened in healthcare. Why not? It seems like such a simple and obvious step! Almost all hospitals and clinics already have some computers. They use them to type letters and send emails, to research on the web and coordinate schedules. They also automate some clinical tasks, most notably medical imaging, which is almost entirely computer-based. But, with few and notable exceptions, clinicians have not computerized the most central information resource they possess, the patient chart. The patient chart remains a paper record, usually a set of papers wrapped in a simple manila envelope.

For most information professionals (or clinical professionals with good information instincts), the use of computers to achieve standardization in data and work processes is a mantra. It is almost beyond question that computerized automation of processes and record-keeping would dramatically improve the performance of any industry. Still, healthcare has resisted computerization for decades.

In the answer to the question "Why hasn't this happened on its own?" we will find the heart of meaningful use. The reasons that healthcare has not computerized can be summarized as screwy incentives and a difficult domain. Specifically:

- Healthcare is orders of magnitude more complex than most other industries. This complexity has generated extensive clinical specialization. In some cases this specialization calls for extensive changes to the "normal" health IT workflow. It also means that each medical specialization has its own diagnostic categories, terminology, and procedures.
- Healthcare is constantly changing. Treatments and best practices that are even two or three years old are frequently so out of date as to be nearly unethical. (Remember Vioxx.)
- Attempts to computerize healthcare facilities have typically failed badly. Many explanations have been offered for this problem, and will be discussed throughout this book.
- Even successful efforts are typically only partial automations, resulting in half-paper and half-computerized workflows that have the benefits of neither system and the drawbacks of both.
- Healthcare providers in the United States, for the most part, are paid for their time. EHR typically slow doctors down, ensuring that they are paid less for the same work.
- Computerization has typically been a very expensive proposition. Healthcare providers have been saddled with this cost, despite the fact that most of the benefits of computerization accrue to either patients or insurers. Essentially, until now, EHR systems have been disincentivized.

These factors, and others like them, have resulted in an abysmal value equation for EHR systems. For the average doctor or hospital, before ARRA funding, buying an EHR system was risky and expensive, with little benefit. To say that adoption of EHR software has been sluggish would be generous. It was widely known that fewer than 20% of small practices in the United States had purchased an EHR before the HITECH act. For a time, conventional wisdom held that although small practices had not purchased EHR systems, they were common (at least over 50%) in hospitals. But a study published in the New England Journal of Medicine in 2009 largely destroyed that illusion.[2] The study compiled a list of the 30 or so tasks that an EHR should do that actually improve the quality of healthcare, and found that less than 10% of all hospitals have installed software that accomplished even a few of these important tasks. The health IT industry was treating EHR deployment as a yes/no question, but if you asked "Is this software actually helping doctors deliver improved care in the hospital?" rather than just "Is something electronic in the hospital?" it became clear that hospital EHR software was typically underperforming.

One of the authors of that study was David Blumenthal. It was not an accident that he was chosen as the National Coordinator for health IT during a critical phase, when

---

2. The Use of Electronic Health Records in U.S. Hospitals (*http://www.rwjf.org/healthpolicy/quality/product.jsp?id=40148*)

meaningful use would first be defined. You might call Dr. Blumenthal an expert in nonmeaningful use.

Health IT in Health Reform

But it is not enough to merely pay doctors to use EHRs. The two counterexamples to systemic failure in health IT are Kaiser Permanente and the VA. The key word here is "systemic," because many other, smaller organizations have succeeded with health IT deployments but they are not comprehensive systems of healthcare. The VA and Kaiser are systems with large numbers of both clinics and hospitals that use advanced health IT systems to effectively coordinate care between locations. Two commonalities between these systems should be mentioned at the outset of any intelligent discussion of perils and potential of health IT.

- Good software that can sustain frequent nimble changes to improve the quality of care
- Financial incentives that encourage improved quality of care rather than merely increased amount of care

This book is all about the first item. Many health associations and experts deal with the second item, but the first must also get our attention for the whole package to work. We will focus on making, deploying, and leveraging good health IT software, but it is useless to think about the purchase and use of EHR software in an environment that disincentivizes those activities. These two concepts form what we call *the VistA effect*, which has turned the VA into the best hospital system in the world. If you do not believe us, I again recommend Longman's book.

Evolution of Meaningful Use

Meaningful use is an attempt by the U.S. government to define the baseline for what a clinician using an EHR should be able to accomplish. But it's not just one set of requirements. Its definition will change every year. It will become more and more stringent as time goes forward, until it encompasses most of what the health IT research community agrees is needed for improved clinical care. Meaningful use is a moving target. The criteria do not explicitly include the deployment of flexible, software that conforms to clinicians' needs as a goal, but without the ability to change gracefully, the same software that meets today's meaningful use requirements will not be able to meet tomorrow's.

Thankfully, meaningful use includes the financial incentives mentioned in the previous section. Its payments occur only when eligible entities prove that they are meaningful users of EHR systems, usually by reporting the details of how they use an EHR system certified for meaningful use. As a result, the meaningful use standards will always focus on specific measurable (and reportable) details of how an EHR system can operate. You need to install a certified system, and use it in valuable ways.

The incentive schedule for HITECH is almost as important as the funds themselves. The ARRA/HITECH incentives are only the beginning. Institutions that adopt systems and use them in certified ways in 2011 and 2012 could getting about $50,000 per doctor in total payments by being meaningful users of certified EHR technology over the period from 2011 to 2016. Those payments could come from either Medicare or Medicaid as bonus payments. Late adopters of the technology get less money, but have the luxury of watching what works among the early EHR adopters. But the real change occurs sometime around 2017. In that year or soon after, Medicare and Medicaid will no longer provide bonus payments for those who have adopted EHR systems, but instead will cut payments to everyone who has not adopted EHR systems. The meaningful use criteria are with us to stay, but the financial process behind meaningful use will serve as carrot for a short time, then it will become a stick.

One of the main limitations of the meaningful use funding is that it applies only to doctors, hospitals, and other eligible providers who bill either Medicaid or Medicare. Taken together, these two programs make the U.S. federal government the largest healthcare purchaser in the United States. But many healthcare providers do not take Medicare or Medicaid at all. There are many more who have threatened to stop taking Medicare or Medicaid if the planned reimbursement cuts are implemented. Many doctors and hospitals will not have the opportunity to get payments under HITECH at all.

But meaningful use will still matter to doctors who forgo Medicare and Medicaid dollars, eventually. Soon after the U.S. federal government starts to penalize healthcare providers who fail to provide EHR-derived healthcare quality data, it is reasonable to assume that private insurance companies will follow suit. In fact this might even happen before then. As soon as EHR systems become pervasive, they will become fair game for discriminatory payments from private insurers. The private insurers in the United States will not join Medicare and Medicaid in paying more for EHRs, but they will certainly join them in paying less for the lack of EHR systems. It is after the bonus payments are entirely gone that meaningful use will truly become a mandate.

Accountable Care Organizations

At the time of this writing, it is hard to predict the course of more fundamental efforts to reform healthcare. The Obama administration has outlined ambitious plans to change the way healthcare in the United States is financed from the ground up. These reform efforts face several legal challenges that will ultimately be resolved by the Supreme Court of the United States, with unforeseeable results.

Not all of these reforms are relevant here, but those that focus on changing healthcare from a system that rewards the *quantity* of care to one that rewards *quality* of care are directly related to meaningful use. Most notable in the evolution of meaningful use is the concept of the accountable care organization (ACO).

ACOs are conceptualized in many different ways, but most of their incarnations focus on capitated or partially capitated care. *Capitation* means that providers are paid a set monthly fee for covered patients, whether they are sick or not. In theory, capitation incentivizes providers to keep patients healthy, thereby reducing the amount of money spent on their healthcare over the long term.

Capitation was at the heart of the health maintenance organization (HMO) movement that began in the United States during the 1970s and continued into the 1980s and 1990s. Eventually HMOs earned a notorious reputation for simply not paying for healthcare to keep costs down. Instead of responding to the incentives in capitation by improving the quality of healthcare delivery, they cut corners and abandoned patients to save money.

What is the difference between the hated HMO model and the currently popular ACO model? Only the capacity to detect whether the care delivered as part of the system is of high quality. The HMO model used statistics to provide models of what treatments were appropriate at given times, and denied treatments that fell outside the model. These simplistic models tended to second-guess healthcare providers about what patients needed, frequently denying coverage for sensible treatments. An ACO, however, should be capable of measuring the end result of a provider's actions to determine whether treatment was successful, making second-guessing unnecessary. An HMO meddled with doctors' methods, whereas an ACO focuses only on the doctors' results. How will an ACO accomplish this? By leveraging data from meaningful use certified EHR systems.

ACOs and concepts like them are an attempt to reform the crazy incentives in healthcare, but those reforms will not work unless it is possible to truly measure the performance of providers through accurate data on the health of the patients in their care. With the data that an EHR provides, an ACO could actively seek out difficult patients, like diabetics, knowing that they would be compensated more for a patient with diabetes. By using smart information systems to customize care, they could treat the diabetic more effectively with lower costs. Everyone wins: the individual diabetic gets better care, the provider gets paid more for providing that care, and the system as a whole pays less for the treatment of that particular diabetic. All of this is made possible by a highly capable EHR system.

In short, meaningful use, paired with the other healthcare reforms, has the potential to initiate the VistA effect, where healthcare organizations constantly measure the quality of care they are delivering and use flexible software to enforce higher and higher levels of patient safety and quality care.

Meaningful use will be at the heart of healthcare reform in the United States for the next several decades, making it one of the most significant components of healthcare reform. To the degree that the United States is a worldwide health IT leader, meaningful use will also have implications internationally.

EHR Functionality in Context

Happily, the meaningful use requirements are relatively short and to the point. The initial version of meaningful use includes features such as demographics, medication list, problem list, and vital signs. These features are trivially intuitive for clinicians, but end up being far more complicated than they seem to implement in software. These core health information constructs become far more complex when we consider just how much we want to do with the underlying data. The first version of meaningful use requires one test of health information exchange, but later versions make it clear that meaningful use will ultimately require providers to securely share patient data with other providers who treat the same patient. Tracking health data and tracking health data in a way compatible with other health data are very different things. Ensuring that health data is liquid is much more complex then just gathering it together.

Things like demographics become tremendously complex in the context of health information exchange. For instance, different healthcare providers in a given city might have electronic records for:

Fred Trotter — 12/31/1975
Frederick Trotter — 12/31/1975
Freddy Trotter — 12/30/1975
Fred Trotten — 12/31/1975

Are these all the same person? If an EHR accepts data sent to it from an outside source, but under a given name that is not the same as one in the EHR database, how should the system react? Should it react differently depending on whether a bill to a insurer under the original given name has been accepted and paid? (Demographic details are a frequent reason for rejection of the payment requests that providers make to third-party payers.) What if the insurance company has the wrong name, but for whatever reason, is unwilling to change it? Do you keep the name you know is wrong for billing purposes, and if so, how do you keep it from polluting data exchange for clinical purposes?

To understand what an item like problem list or demographics truly means in terms of EHR systems, you have to understand a tremendous amount of healthcare-related context, as well as a few sticky points of software design. Things in healthcare IT often work counterintuitively to the normal workings of IT. This is because things in healthcare work very differently than in any other industry. The issues associated with medical billing alone are usually enough upend typical IT approaches. At the end of this book you should be able to read the meaningful use requirements and have an understanding of what it will take to execute them. You should be able to recognize which issues in health IT are open, difficult problems, and which issues have already been solved by industry best practices. You will be able to see through those pundits who frequently present health IT molehills as mountains or mountains as molehills. We also believe that you will begin to see the meaningful use requirements just as we do: a reasonable set of standards that are simple enough to actually fulfill, with enough punch to still make a difference in healthcare. Like many health IT experts, your authors can tend to be jaded, but we see the meaningful use requirements as fundamental evidence of good government. It is difficult to strike any kind of balance with health IT standards and the Office of the National Coordinator has done a good job of this with the meaningful use requirements.

It has taken software professionals about a decade to get up to speed on health IT, a decade that was frequently spent in confusion and frustration. We remain confused and frustrated with health IT. The authors still think, however, this industry also holds the highest hopes for IT: to make a real difference in peoples lives. We have seen far too many IT professionals leave health IT because the frustrations with the daily grind outweighed the hope for change. We believe that by reading this book, you can skip part of that process that we went through, and be confused, frustrated, and hopeful at a much higher level.

CHAPTER 2

An Anatomy of Medical Practice

"When you've seen one medical practice, you've seen
one medical practice."

We can't think of an expression that better embodies the difficulties of understanding medical operations than the one heading this chapter. Regardless of how much a facility might think it embodies the "typical operations" and "common practices" respective to the lines of care it delivers and region in which it is located, our collective experience finds few if any typical operations and common practices exist. This diversity is frequently true of facilities even in the same buildings and campuses.

A quick look at the market share of various technological systems sheds light on the variety of software and hardware out there. The largest vendor in EHR systems holds only a self-reported 12% of the market by provider count and 16% by patient count. If you contrast that with operational software in every other major industry, healthcare is extremely fragmented with respect to IT. The authors aren't aware of any research that fully explains the reasons for fragmentation, but market forces in healthcare are very different from those in other industries. It is possible to speculate that because institutions that might be forced to close in other industries are sustained by many different forces manipulating the market in healthcare, the longevity of intact facilities is much longer compared to an industry such as retail. That longevity is a barrier to change and leads to fragmentation.

So where does that leave us? Although there is not a single simple picture that can be painted of medical operations, we can take a tour of the variety of roles, departments, and operations that come together to form practices or hospitals. There does exist one clear line that can be drawn in looking at operations and that line is the distinction between *outpatient* and *inpatient* services, so that is where we will start.

There is an important distinction between inpatient and outpatient terms as they apply to this book. *Inpatient* facilities we define as those that treat patients primarily in 24-hour cycles or fractions thereof. *Outpatient* facilities we define as treating patients primarily in distinct visits. A visit could be only a few minutes or could run most of a day.

Whether a certain facility is inpatient or not can come down to some very fine hair-splitting and brings to mind the "you know it when you see it" standard sometimes applied in the law with respect to obscenity cases. To be a literal hospital or not to be a hospital is often a financially driven decision made by the organization and how they would like to be categorized by various agencies and regulators. So in this text we are going to dodge that particular issue and focus on a slightly different one. Although the name of this chapter mentions the anatomy of a hospital, what we actually mean is the anatomy of *inpatient* care. Outpatient is defined here as care where the interaction with the patient is episodic, and inpatient is where the patient is treated continuously in small increments of time regularly running over several 24-hour cycles.

There do exist some similarities between the operations at outpatient and inpatient facilities but for the most part they operate in distinct ways. Those distinctions are noted throughout the following overview of their operations.

Going back to terminology, we can introduce the terms *visits* or *encounters*, which outpatient facilities use interchangeably to refer to their interactions with patients. Outpatient facilities tend to refer to their visits or encounters as occurring in numbers of exam rooms. For inpatient facilities they refer to the intake of their patients as *admissions* or *admits* and refer to the locations as *beds* and *numbers of beds*, referring in most cases to actual physical beds in the facility.

How Patients Reach Healthcare Organizations

The first thing to understand about medical operations is how patients find their way to them. We can then examine the different elements that make up most organizations. Patients reach outpatient sites in two fundamental ways. They might begin contact themselves after hearing about the practice from a friend or from a listing on the Internet or in an insurance directory. They might have also been referred to the facility by another doctor or social support organization.

The way that patients find themselves coming to an *inpatient* facility is usually not a positive one. It most often means that the patient has an acute condition or trauma and has come in via an Emergency Department (ER), has received a diagnosis from an outpatient facility that required more investigation or a complex treatment or surgery, has a complex condition or chronic condition that he or she has self-identified as being best handled by an inpatient facility, or that he or she is choosing to have an elective procedure performed that can only be done on an inpatient basis.

As a general rule of thumb the smallest inpatient facility is bigger than the smallest medical practice. The smallest inpatient facility that comes to mind is an eight-bed facility focusing on mental health, known within healthcare as behavioral health. It is much more common to see inpatient facilities from 15–65 beds, considered small, and from 65–250 beds, considered medium and large. There are a few select facilities in the United States that are bigger still. Those facilities run by counties or the VA are often much, much larger, commonly called mega-hospitals or super-hospitals. They tend to function a bit more like a city than a typical medical organization and won't be covered in this text.

In outpatient care, when the contact is initiated by the patient, the *front office* receives the phone call or Internet contact and determines whether that new patient is an appropriate fit for the facility. That fit is based on a variety of factors and the type of care and problems they need to have addressed. One type of contact almost all of us are familiar with is a sick visit or flu follow-up. Often we visit a different physician than our primary provider because of the immediacy of the need. Outpatient organizations that specialize in same-day visits are usually called urgent care facilities, and tend not to see patients on an ongoing basis. These facilities commonly establish a general time the patient can show up as an unscheduled walk-in visit rather than requiring the patient to make a formal appointment. Sometimes they might even use a take-a-number approach instead of a more traditional appointment.

Within this initial transaction between a facility and patient we have to consider the myriad of specialties and types of facilities that exist in the United States. The spectrum of care is enormous from sites such as Federally Qualified Health Centers (FQHC), which have a mandate to treat everyone regardless of insurance, to specialty medicine sites like oncology (cancer medicine), dialysis, HIV/AIDS care, pain management, pediatrics, and geriatrics, to elective care such as dermatology. The federal government recognizes about 240 specialties for outpatient care, but practically speaking there are thousands. For inpatient care there are roughly 100 official categorizations, but again, in practice there are easily 1,000 or more. Like we said at the start of this chapter, "When you've seen one medical practice, you've seen one medical practice."

With inpatient care there are small hospitals specializing in particular areas of surgery, general institutions serving a wide range of needs for a geographical area, institutions like the VA that service only a unique subset of the patient population, trauma centers that handle the most difficult and serious injuries in a region, and long-term care that services patients who require continuous assistance for a few weeks to several months or years. Those are just the types that immediately come to mind.

Based on the type of care, there are many considerations in how the appointment might be made. Whether an appointment is necessary at all and how long it might be before the patient is able to actually come to the site and be seen vary from case to case. A shockingly large percentage of *outpatient* facilities still keep their appointments in paper appointment books or rudimentary electronic systems such as spreadsheets and online calendars. Although meaningful use does not have a specific requirement for tracking appointments electronically it is convenient for vendors to implement such support because of other guideline requirements. In addressing the rest of the requirements, all systems that are meaningful use certified include some amount of scheduling features and generally include a comprehensive scheduling module.

Appointments for new patients at outpatient sites typically begin with obtaining information. At a minimum that might consist of a name, phone number, and general reason regarding the visit. In referral cases where the patient is coming from another facility a summary record or a comprehensive record will be faxed or couriered and is a precondition before the patient is actually seen. Things begin to get complicated quickly as we talk about other preconditions for an actual visit and all the pieces that need to be in place before a patient can be seen by a provider.

Before most scheduled visits, laboratory tests on blood or other fluids need to be conducted with sufficient time for the results to be completed before the provider visit. Because labs themselves often require billing and other administrative operations, there is practically speaking "a visit" before the scheduled provider visit.

Inpatient scheduling has some additional complexity beyond that found in outpatient centers because of coordinated staffing needs including many more personnel and because of physical resource availability. Outpatient facilities are usually scaled to handle more than their normal operating capacity and have constraints mostly based on single personnel. Inpatient systems are more complex because most, if not all, procedures will involve several personnel, including a surgeon or procedure technician, an anesthesiologist, specially trained surgical or scrub nurses, and personnel to handle the patient post-surgery. Even for nonsurgical treatments, a senior provider, one or more technicians, and nurses and orderlies might be involved.

Most inpatient procedures also involve very expensive equipment and operating rooms, which can severely constrain the number of procedures that can occur in a particular time frame. For example, many orthopedic surgeries require specific operating tools that are expensive and in limited supply, so even if a facility had the staff and operating room available they would not be able to perform two hip replacements at that same time. They might even need several hours between procedures due to the time of the procedure, the time to assess the equipment before and after use for safety and operation, and the need to sterilize the equipment for use again.

Further complicating inpatient scheduling at facilities with an emergency room is the general unpredictability of those needs. That unpredictability results in the frequent rescheduling of elective procedures at sites running above about 50% of their overall capacity. It also results in the scheduling of elective procedures during very early morning hours that statistically coincide with the least busy time for accidents and traumas. Although scheduling is primarily at the discretion of the performing providers, it is not helpful to anyone to have unpredictable rescheduling, so it is best avoided.

Taking into account those factors, inpatient scheduling is not wholly different from outpatient scheduling and both assign people and equipment to be allocated to particular patients' needs over the course of their admission or visit to the facility.

Lab Sample Collection Before a Visit or Admission Date

Although it might not seem an obvious fit, the next step after scheduling and before an actual visit or admission takes place is most often the collection of samples for lab tests. Depending on the type of visit scheduled, lab sample collection might be done at the practice or hospital or at a third-party lab service center run by a large lab company or a nearby regional hospital that offers third-party lab services. The results then come back via fax or electronically via a website. Most facilities complete only the sample collection, such as drawing blood (known as phlebotomy) on the outpatient side, with only very large multipractice groups operating their own full-service laboratories that perform the actual tests. Samples get collected in one place and sent to another for the actual testing. Samples are picked up by the performing lab on a daily basis, but results can take from a day or two to more than a week.

The lab sample collection area is the location where patients, typically on a walk-in but sometimes on a scheduled basis, come to have blood, urine, and stool samples collected. The specific collections are based on the orders from the provider involved. Having the results is usually prerequisite information before the outpatient visit or inpatient admission can occur. At inpatient sites of even modest size, the tests on the samples are performed on site and results are computed for the majority of tests. They can then be viewed in an electronic system or provided on paper. Meaningful use dictates that results, at a minimum, be received electronically for the majority of tests.

Most of the time the lab sample collection for routine lab tests happens about two weeks before the visit or admission. Obviously in trauma settings or any urgent case that lead time isn't always possible and rush labs are done. If the situation dictates, results can be obtained sometimes within just a few minutes for chemical tests. Tests that require the culture of bacteria cannot be rushed because it takes time for the cultures to grow and multiply.

HIPAA and Patient Identification

Once a patient arrives for her visit or admission a number of forms and several types of information are gathered. This is where a commonly misunderstood and misquoted set of laws and regulations meet squarely with the real world. The law we are referring to is the Health Insurance Portability and Accountability Act (HIPAA). We discuss some important specifics in Chapter 12, while covering the broad scope here.

The first purpose and practice of HIPAA is to regulate the dissemination of data collected in healthcare interactions. That aspect is commonly referred to as the Privacy Rule. HIPAA additionally defines standards of operation an organization must take to restrict access to the information it tracks and stores. This is commonly referred to as the Security Rule. The HITECH act of 2009, which was part of the overall stimulus legislation, amended HIPAA to more specifically address details on handling medical information in the Internet age.

The first form a new patient will complete is almost always a HIPAA Authorization. Sometimes this is called a HIPAA waiver, even though that is a bit of a misnomer. This form clarifies the details of distribution and grants permission to the treating organization to disseminate the medical information in specific ways needed for treatment to occur. In certain scenarios it might also authorize dissemination to specific third parties such as lab organizations, imaging (X-ray, MRI, etc.) centers, and contracted or referring doctors and specialists.

Next is the medical consent for treatment and the consent for billing, which is often combined into a single agreement. The billing consent permits the treating organization to work with the patient's insurance company on his or her behalf to cover costs for treatment. It usually requires the patient to guarantee that any costs not covered by the insurance company will become the responsibility of the patient.

The medical consent is the basic permission the practice needs to collect vital statistics such as blood pressure, collect specimens for labs such as a blood draw, and conduct other broad interactions with the patient that might otherwise constitute assault under the law. It also indicates that patients assume a level of decision making and responsibility for their own care. Patients are obligated to provide comprehensive details about known allergies, existing medications, and both personal and family medical history. If you know you have a severe allergy to penicillin-based antibiotics and forget to disclose that, the practice is not usually liable for malpractice if you are prescribed one and have an adverse reaction.

Specific or complex procedures or those that have particular health risks or potential side effects will have separate consents that a medical provider will review with the patient directly. Those are unique to each case and distinct from the general medical consent for treatment we are discussing here.

We touched on this when talking about scheduling but it is worth repeating. A shockingly large number of outpatient facilities are still using paper-based appointment books, spreadsheets, or various online calendars. Unfortunately all three of those methods are unlikely to comply with the HIPAA privacy and security rules. Although HIPAA was initiated in 1996, it was not until 2011 that there began to be serious enforcement action by the federal government, fining facilities that are not compliant. Replacing those noncompliant systems should be a priority for any new implementation of any meaningful use system.

Management and acceptance of risk plays a significant role in the workflow of inpatient facilities in a process referred to as *informed consent*. Outpatient care is generally concerned only with general consent for treatment that broadly outlines common risks and interventions. Inpatient facilities are required to provide the patient with a specific understanding of the procedure to be performed, the risks and potential outcomes if the procedure is completed, and the risks and potential outcomes if the procedure is not completed. Patients then have to make their own personal decision about whether those risks are acceptable.

It is absolutely vital that inpatient facilities properly document the patient's understanding and acceptance of a specific intervention's risks or face tremendous liability if something goes wrong. As a result, much administrative overhead is spent documenting, educating, and tracking the consents. The informed consents are often handled by the provider in concert with the billing personnel collecting the information from the patients or their responsible parties.

With consents out of the way it is necessary to confront the issue of patient identification. This is an enormously complex problem that can result in severe or fatal adverse events when mistakes are made. The most conscientious facilities and systems will utilize a combination of name, date of birth, primary identification number (such as a Social Security number), and an identification picture. The combination of those data points is used to confirm that a particular person is in fact the same one in the selected medical record.

Care must be taken not to confuse patients with the same name or date of birth or cases where both of those data points match across multiple people. Many facilities commonly search for or identify patients by date of birth alone. Unfortunately, this practice is statistically dangerous and advised against in the most recent guidelines from several data standards organizations (HITSP and NIST).

A scenario known to statisticians that relates is called the *birthday problem*, which states there is a 99% chance that 2 people in a group of 57 will share an exact birthdate. In practice the odds are even more likely for specific dates relating to holidays and their association with births. When you take the example of prevalent names such as Smith, Jones, or Hernandez and the volume of patients at even small facilities, it is absolutely essential that cases with patients sharing the same name and date of birth be specifically trained for and protected against. This is best done by a third confirmation of a primary identifier such as a Social Security number or insurance policy number and a patient picture.

With a patient properly identified, the paper record is either created for new patients or found for existing patients. Where possible an organization will pull patient records from their storage area into a staging area based on patients who are scheduled to be seen. This reduces wait times when patients arrive but presents an additional stage during which identification mistakes can be made.

Within a site, a numeric or alphanumeric identifier is assigned and in the case of paper records is applied with stickers to the paper folder containing the record documents. This identifier is typically called the *medical record number* (MRN). For organizations with multiple locations or departments it isn't uncommon for a single patient to be assigned multiple MRNs. Each department operating separately assigns its own unique MRN to the same person. This can present a problem once records become electronic, as there will be multiple numbers referring to the same patient.

In the electronic world it is a fundamental benefit that information can be quickly and seamlessly shared between respective parties. That benefit leads to our first general rule of EHR and MU implementation: one patient, one record number. If an allergy or medication is recorded on an electronic record it is instantly visible in another. If multiple records with distinct record numbers exist for the same physical person they will need to be merged or linked, or else crucial information can be fragmented and missed.

Intake, Demographics, Visits, and Admissions

Demographics data about the patient might or might not be collected in current workflows. This data includes race, ethnicity, education level, primary language, and a few other characteristics that are specified by meaningful use criteria. Today a relatively small percentage of practices collect all that information but it plays a crucial role in determining overall efficacy of treatments and availability of services in particular regions. Meaningful use requires a specific set of demographics data be collected for compliance and this will be a new activity for many organizations not use to the level of detail required.

For most inpatient procedures there is an additional set of steps patients must follow before they actually arrive for admission. This can be as simple as forgoing food 12 hours before surgery to reduce potential complications from anesthesia, or as complex as detailed drug regimens to affect an ailment so that it can be addressed once admittance occurs. In inpatient care, the coordination of these activities is normally handled by the admissions department or what is sometimes called the outreach department.

With the demographics collection and intake paperwork completed there is almost always an interaction with a nurse, medical assistant, or physician assistant. Those personnel are often known as midlevel providers, which distinguishes them from the medical doctors and family nurse practitioners who can prescribe and act as the legal treating providers of record. The midlevels collect information about allergies and current medications, and qualify the reason for the visit or admission. Depending on circumstances, personal as well as family medical history might be taken, although the specifics vary based on the line of care or procedure scheduled.

That information gathering is then followed by necessary physical information gathering, which encompasses vital statistics including height, weight, systolic and diastolic blood pressure, beats per minute, respirations per minute, and pulse oximetry. In an inpatient setting additional samples for lab tests might be taken for immediate processing and results received before the procedure is done. Other specialties or specific cases will require collection of additional information such as peak flow respirations for asthmatics or analyzing height and weight growth for pediatrics.

The most straightforward type of interaction a patient might have at an inpatient facility is an *elective* or *precautionary* minor surgery or minor procedure. We will start with that scenario to explain the inpatient care workflow, but will cover several other common interactions as well. If you opt to have a surgery that is not trauma related, or is something that could be delayed without adverse medical consequence, it is considered an elective procedure.

A common example of an elective procedure is something like an orthopedic surgery, perhaps a hip replacement. Another might be a cosmetic surgery. A hip replacement is usually considered necessary because of pain or limitation to mobility but it can also be delayed for weeks or even months because a later timing does not usually present significant medical risks to the patient. Some things like preventative colonoscopy can also be found in inpatient settings and are done on an elective scheduled basis rather than emergency one.

Precertification and Prior Authorization

For very expensive procedures such as chemotherapy in the treatment of cancer or outpatient procedures, organizations work directly with insurance companies before the activity actually takes place. This coordination is a process known as *precertification*. Precertification can provide a level of certainty to the treating organization that the procedure will be paid for by the patient's insurance company before it is actually performed. Precertification results in a special authorization code that must appear in the billing documents for the patient.

At inpatient facilities this is typically called *prior authorization*. Practically speaking this is not much different from precertification. This step is normally done for elective and scheduled procedures and also plays a role in drug selection and imaging studies. For traumas and other emergency treatment, time does not permit this step, nor does a lack of insurance disqualify the patient from having the treatment. Under the law, although you can be billed for whatever activities an inpatient site performs on you, if you are at immediate risk of death or severe disability the facility is obligated to provide you treatment regardless of your financial or insurance situation. At large facilities, prior authorization will often be its own department. At smaller and medium-sized sites, it is often combined with the billing department.

Emergency Admissions

Now that we have discussed how patients who are scheduled arrive at inpatient facilities we can look at how unscheduled patients arrive. The main avenue through which patients unexpectedly need inpatient care is through the emergency department (ER). There is also a class of patients who might be in need of inpatient care on an urgent but not quite emergency basis. Patients facing imminent risk of severe injury or death, known as morbidity (injury) and mortality (death), can be considered as *trauma* patients. They need immediate medical intervention or risk permanent disability or even death. Patients who are facing a serious or potentially life-threatening condition but who might have some amount of time for their care to be coordinated are known as *acute* cases.

The first course of action in emergency care is determining the relative priority of patients in a process called *triage*, which is discussed in more detail later. With that determination, available resources are allocated accordingly. The *sickest* patients receive the most immediate attention.

Trauma care typically involves four primary medical *interventions*: the administration of drugs, application of life support, surgery, and nonsurgical procedures. A nonsurgical procedure might be something such as cardiac catheterization to relieve clogged arteries. Many patients will receive more than one of those types of interventions during the course of their treatment. After the trauma is resolved the patient is introduced to either a standard room and bed or an intensive care unit (ICU) if he or she remains critical or unstable and requires constant supervision and attention.

A common example of a *trauma* patient would be a car accident patient who has internal bleeding from the violent impact of the crash. Unless the bleeding is stopped with an immediate surgery the patient is likely to die very quickly and the longer the wait the more the odds for survival decrease.

A common example of an *acute* patient would be someone who has suffered a heart attack. The patient has been stabilized but needs a heart surgery such as a coronary bypass before he or she can be released. That patient might be kept reasonably healthy and stable while in the hospital but would be at severe risk for further disability or death if he or she tried to return to normal life without treatment. For reasons of cost control and improved outcomes, the patient is typically scheduled for treatment within days rather than on an emergency basis. Scheduling can also depend on the availability of the resources as we have already discussed.

The fundamental point to take away from the difference between *trauma* and *acute* care is the balancing of risk. Not eating 12 hours before a surgery reduces the risks of certain known complications from anesthesia. However if the condition of the patient is so severe he or she isn't likely to survive long without further injury or death then the fact that he or she has just eaten dinner before the accident becomes an acceptable risk.

In regard to information technology, acute and trauma care present the most challenging environment and bring a weighty importance to the notion of a mission-critical system. Failure or a degradation in performance of such a system can result in the injury or death of a patient in a very direct way not common in most other IT. It is absolutely imperative that the worst case scenarios be accounted for, including power loss, network failures, and many other events with suitable alternative workflows. Several states such as California also have legislation that requires specific steps to mitigate the risks to patients in those scenarios.

Prioritization and Triage

Starting with the emergency department, we come to one of the crucial logistical considerations that play a major role in inpatient care and another complicating factor that has some impact on outpatient care as well. That consideration is *triage*, or the need to prioritize certain patients because of their condition. That prioritization then leads to treatments that achieve the best outcome for all of the patients present rather than only looking at a single case.

An overly simplistic example of triage is how an elective procedure that can be rescheduled with mild inconvenience will be postponed due to something like the internal bleeding surgery we discussed in the last section. That would cause the elective surgery to be bumped from an operating room so the high-priority surgery could take place first. In more real-world and complex scenarios the prioritization depends heavily on the judgment and experience of the providers involved.

A commonly heard term in hospital settings on TV is the word STAT. This word actually comes from the Latin *statim*, meaning immediately. It is in some sense the determination once triage has been conducted. An action flagged as STAT should jump the queue and move to the front of the line with respect to conducting lab tests, administering medication, or a variety of other activities. Although the literal STAT is used to some extent in hospital settings it is more common to see a set of four or five unique priority levels that determine the sequence in which activities are handled. This notion of jumping the queue can wreak havoc on carefully thought-out or orchestrated workflows.

One of the deceptively complex areas for managing triage involves imaging. Most hospitals have a resource constraint when it comes to MRI, CAT scans, and other types of complex imaging. Frequently more patients have imaging needs than a facility has machines available. Because these machines are typically used in diagnosis rather than treatment, scheduling them is a very complicated endeavor. A patient might have been in an auto accident, appear with only minor injuries, but need an MRI to make a determination about a head injury.

Should that patient take precedence over another that has an MRI scheduled before a planned surgery?

Those tough types of judgment calls result in ripples and delays throughout the hospital workflow that make logistics difficult to manage efficiently and are a unique type of challenge facing the transition to more electronic systems.

Outpatient Care

Meaningful use places a particular importance on vital statistics including blood pressure, height, weight, pulse, respiration, and pulse oximetry (oxygenation of the blood). In some settings it has not been considered necessary to collect all these details, or maybe they weren't done on every visit. Meaningful use with limited exceptions requires their collection on every new encounter with the patient. The motivating factor for collecting this information routinely is its strong correlation with preventing acute or trauma incidents.

A visit to a dermatologist who collects those vitals could prevent a trip to the ER if an undiagnosed and problematically high blood pressure or other strong risk factor is found. Each interaction with a medical professional becomes a basic screening for the most widespread risk factors. When performed on a large scale, this can reduce costs in the system as a whole and increase positive outcomes for patients. Those two factors are really the motivations that brought about meaningful use.

From a terminology standpoint the people who interact with patients regarding clinical issues can be collectively referred to as *providers*. That term encompasses all of the acronym soup that persons delivering primary treatment might be accredited with. Typically nurses or other midlevel staff are not referred to as providers but that can vary depending on the primacy of their role in a particular treatment.

With the vitals and related information gathering completed the patient is handed off to the actual provider. From state to state and in different lines of care, that provider could be a family nurse practitioner (FNP), a physician assistant (PA), a doctor of osteopathic medicine (DO), or the more familiar medical doctor (MD). For the most part in most states all of those just listed can prescribe, diagnose conditions, and order treatments. Prescribing medications that are regulated by the Drug Enforcement Agency (DEA), such as strong painkillers like Vicodin, might be limited to only DO and MD providers. This is excepted in some jurisdictions in a very complicated area of the law.

Providers' interactions vary tremendously based on the line of care they practice so we will walk through what is known as the *general practice* interaction. That is the type of visit most of us are familiar with. Everything from a doctor's visit because of the flu to an annual physical falls into the general practice category. We will also briefly cover some common specialties of medicine.

The most common method of operating today for general practice is known as the Subjective, Objective, Assessment, Plan Model (SOAP). It is the typical means of operating in most general practices, but not all. SOAP also has applicability to a large number of specialties. Simply put SOAP is a model for documenting the interaction with the patient that brings some repeatability, consistency, and quality controls to how the interaction is conducted. Even though each patient's circumstances and needs can be extremely unique, SOAP helps add a structure that produces a similar result for a similar interaction.

In addition to or as part of SOAP, the provider must also record procedure codes and diagnostic codes to bill the visit to an insurance program or other funding source. We'll cover a lot more about those codes in Chapter 3. In a paper world these codes are typically recorded on a sheet called a superbill or an encounter form. The form consists of a preselected list of codes that can be easily checked off.

Once completed, the superbill ends up with the billing department, where its information is entered into an electronic system. A system used specifically for billing is often known as a *practice management system*. Some vendors offer a combined EHR and practice management system. Some practices do the data entry of codes via internal staff, a biller or coder. Others send the paper out to be handled by a third party known as a billing service that does the data entry.

Whole books and courses cover the specific practice of SOAP, but from a technology standpoint it can be understood as an organizational breakdown of mostly text and narrative that the provider uses to record an interaction with the patient. It starts with the subjective discussion of the patient's problems and reason for the visit, which can encompass acute issues like a cold or flu as well as chronic problems such as pain, asthma, or diabetes. The provider will then revise and assess the needs of the patient and create the plan, which might consist of patient instructions, prescriptions, lab tests, referral orders, procedure orders, follow-up visits, and instructions for other staff.

With the SOAP process and coding process completed, the patient might be able to exit the practice entirely, return to the lab technician (phlebotomist) for additional sample collection, visit with a nurse or case worker for referral or other follow-up, or reach an administrative desk for discharge and payment.

Meaningful use requires the patient to be able to receive a summary of his or her visit in a timely manner, which should include the charges and codes. This represents a major change for many practices that are accustomed to taking much longer to supply the patient with that information.

Inpatient Care

Care inside an inpatient workflow can be infinitely complex. In some cases there is the planned reason the patient is being admitted to the facility but then there is the reaction and re-reaction to complications or other factors encountered during the planned treatment. Trauma cases are by their very definition unpredictable.

Surgery is a common intervention that involves several different subdepartments operating in concert with each other to function smoothly. Prior to surgery patients will undergo preparations involving the administration of pre-anesthesia drugs and sedatives, physical preparation such as shaving or marking areas relevant to the surgery, application of imaging technology for use during the surgery, and communication about how events will proceed.

During the surgery, surgeons work with a team of staff including monitoring nurses and other staff who are responsible for watching certain vital statistics and data during the procedure and communicating with parties outside the operating room, scrub nurses and other assistants who support the surgeons, and the anesthesiologist who is responsible for administering and monitoring the patient's anesthesia and respiratory functions.

Immediately following the completion of a surgery a stable patient will be moved to the post-anesthesia care unit (PACU). The PACU is responsible for seeing that the patient is able to come off life support that might have been applied during the surgery, administering pain management medications as well as prophylactic measures, and monitoring for complications. Finally the PACU will communicate with patients as they regain consciousness.

At each step of the way all of the activities, supplies, and events occurring with the patient are documented in several forms that involve paperwork, dictation, and in some cases direct computer entry. Those records wend their way to the billing department for disposition into claims. Those claims represent units of time, typically in 15-minute increments as well as individual line items for each unit of drug, unit of supply, and unit of personnel involved in the care.

It is not uncommon for certain charges to be highlighted as outrageous, such as the infamous $10 aspirin. Although there are cases where overcharging for certain items is done to cover costs for other unrelated care at a facility, in most cases the time of nonprovider personnel cannot be billed directly and is lumped into supply and medication costs. The overhead staff costs are rolled into the supply cost for something like aspirin. Administration of that aspirin involved an order from a provider, dispensing from a pharmacy, administration by a nurse, and all the associated record-keeping and auditing of each of those steps.

Hospitals differ from outpatient facilities in that typically contain both an on-premises pharmacy and an on-premises lab. The precise extent of each of those depends greatly on the types of procedures done at the facility. At institutions with more than 40 or 50 beds, facilities will most often have fully comprehensive labs and pharmacies on site. The ordering and fulfillment of activities at those on-site centers varies greatly with some acting as tightly integrated departments of the overall facility and some acting as semi-independent silos with distinct systems, management, and operations.

In summarizing the differences between inpatient and outpatient care, we find that inpatient care is primarily centered around small and continuous increments of time, whereas outpatient care is centered around transactional visits or encounters with the patient. Inpatient care typically operates on a larger scale, with many services and types of care contained within a single facility's walls, whereas outpatient facilities depend more on partnerships and referrals to outside parties.

Labs

Some larger practices will conduct almost all of the lab tests themselves in an on-premises laboratory. We could easily spend another chapter on that but for sake of brevity we will highlight just the most important points. Labs operate typically with another electronic system (LIMS or laboratory information system) distinct from the EHR or by a paper process different from the medical practice itself. They are governed and licensed by distinct regulations and requirements collectively referred to as CLIA.

At a lab appointment prior to the provider visit or at the actual provider visit, a number of important administrative steps should be performed so that the visit can be appropriately billed to an insurance company or other funding program with the patient's consent to work with his or her insurer. It is critical that the patient can be properly identified, that his or her privacy preferences are respected, and that the patient provides informed medical consent for treatment.

Lab tests themselves are for the most part performed by automated robotic machines. Automated machines are used for commonly ordered lab tests contained in the Comprehensive Metabolic Panel (CMP) or Comprehensive Blood Count (CBC). You have almost certainly had those done on a recent visit to the doctor; they detail the basic chemistry of your blood and quantify its biological functioning. It is possible to perform those tests manually but it is rare.

Microbiology and culture tests are still done manually in most labs but more and more are moving to robotic systems as well. Pathology is for the most part still manual but certain tests such as a PAP smear have automated systems available. Automated systems for microbiology and pathology tend to be prohibitively expensive.

When tests are ordered by the provider they can be ordered individually but it is much faster and more common for them to be ordered as a named group. Those groups are called *panels*, two of which were just mentioned. A very common one, the CBC, is a set of tests including a white blood cell count, a red blood cell count, and so forth. The most common scenario for the performing laboratory is that orders come in as panels and results go out as individual test results organized in groupings that might or might not reflect how they were ordered.

Imaging

At small- and medium-sized practices the only common imaging equipment located on site is an individual X-ray machine and an ultrasound machine. For many types of imaging studies a radiologist, a medical doctor solely specialized in examining imaging results, is legally needed to interpret the images. Having that person on staff all the time is not feasible for many small and medium-sized sites to justify based on volume.

For basic X-rays, a regular doctor can in some states make determinations to diagnose pneumonia and certain bone fractures, although at increased risk of malpractice. That is found typically at small or rural practices where a comprehensive imaging center is not readily available. If any ambiguity remains about the result the practice will refer the results for further review by an off-site radiologist or send the patient to a comprehensive imaging center for an additional study.

Ultrasound is common in many small practices and used very commonly in OB/GYN care. It is a relatively inexpensive and small device with fairly straightforward results. It can also be a very profitable activity for small practices to do on site as reimbursements by insurance carriers and Medicare are fairly generous for the amount of work and equipment it actually requires.

Administration and Billing

With most of the clinical aspects of a practice reviewed we can focus on the administrative and billing part of the workflow. Without billing, the majority of medical practices cannot operate, so it is the heart of most site's workflows. Billing operations at medical practices also constitute the most complex workflows of any activity in any industry and we don't say that lightly. I had the husband of a doctor who started a small three-provider medical practice once tell me that he "Could not wrap his head around the billing operations, they just didn't make any sense." He was the nuclear safety officer and engineer for a U.S. Navy carrier battle group.

The way billing for medical services operates today is the result of a bizarre nexus of market incentives and disincentives, more than 70 years of legislative schizophrenia, and the fundamental tension of the U.S. healthcare system. That fundamental tension is that we are a very sick nation, mostly self-inflicted, but as a result necessary care costs more than most patients can afford. Chapter 3 is dedicated in more detail to billing, but here we review the basic outline of the workflow.

The codes selected by the providers during the interaction with the patient need to be cleaned up according to very complex rules and procedures defined by insurers or programs such as Medicare. They are then priced according to a number of factors relating to the patient, the insurance carrier, and the specifics of the practice. Then those codes are bundled up into an electronic or paper submission and sent to either the insurer or a third-party middle man known as a clearinghouse that sends them on to the insurer.

Practices still on a paper workflow might have an additional middle man known as a billing service that performs the cleaning up and data entry tasks for them. Those submissions are known as a claim.

The payer receives the claim and based on more complex rules refuses to accept it, denies it, or pays most but typically not all of the money that was billed. That payer returns a complex document known as an explanation of benefits (EOB) that defines on a code-by-code basis what was paid, what was not paid, and categorical reasons why. That EOB winds its way back through the middle man and is either electronically imported or manually entered into the practice management system for review by the billing department.

For claims that are not accepted or are denied by the insurance, the practice typically has the option to correct information and resubmit. Depending on the insurance companies and their rules, denials and refusals can occur due to extremely benign things relating to patient demographic information, from something as simple as a missing middle initial on the patient's insurance policy to cases where the procedure is not covered at all by insurance or insurance has lapsed or is no longer active.

Many patients receive insurance from multiple carriers that each might cover only a portion of the activities performed by the provider. It is the responsibility of the billing department to coordinate the transmission of the claim to all the relevant insurers and to then follow up on any remaining balances with the patient or person financially responsible for the patient.

Billing departments, because of their importance, are also typically the administrative center of a practice and do the bulk of operational reporting. For the most part, reporting is typical of most service businesses and looks at the breakdowns of which types of services were provided, efficiency and utilization of those services, and the financial aspects of costs versus revenue.

Meaningful use opens up several avenues of complex reporting about specific clinical benchmarks that will be new ground to most practices. The purpose of this reporting is to identify specific details about the most problematic and common diseases centering around diabetes, hypertension, asthma, and high cholesterol. Before the use of EHR at facilities it has been extremely time consuming and expensive to perform basic analysis such as determining what percentage of the patients seen last year have diabetes, or what percentage of diabetics seen were effectively controlling their blood sugar. Although these questions seem very basic, it has been only recently with the onset of EHR systems that they can be looked at on a large scale.

Once patients are leaving the practice they might be coordinated for future visits at the current site or for visits to outside facilities to which they are being referred. Outside referrals are often for the purposes of imaging, lab testing, or consultation by a different provider or specialist.

CHAPTER 3

Medical Billing

Medical billing in the United States ranks, in our experience, with nuclear physics and rocket design in challenges to mastery. These fields all have incredibly steep learning curves and require years of study, patience, and experience. We are not joking about this. Medical billing is one of the most difficult tasks that can be undertaken, and performing it successfully is an extraordinary feat. The United States generates more than $3 trillion of medical spending per year, which leaves the payers (insurance, government, patients) in an all-out war to avoid paying as much as they can to the recipients such as facilities, providers, and other servicers. To put that $3 trillion number in perspective for a moment, realize that the entire federal government across all operations, including defense, spends just a little more than $3 trillion per year. Healthcare is the largest pie out there, but it is exceptionally hard to get a slice.

Between terminology, legal issues, coding, and the mechanics of claims, this chapter has an enormous amount of material to cover, so be prepared to stick around for a while. We will provide a good overview of medical billing workflows as well as a Rosetta stone for the jargon you are likely to encounter. Understand, however, that even with this chapter's length we can only begin to scratch the surface of all that medical billing entails. Medicare alone, the federal government insurer, has more than 2 million pages of documentation describing the rules, regulations, and mechanics of billing only that organization. We don't want to dishearten you further, but there are more than 2,000 payer organizations in the United States, each with voluminous and conflicting sets of regulations.

Starting off, it is important to identify a couple of quick terms that will make explaining a lot of workflow steps more concise. First, we use *the system* to refer to healthcare as a whole: all activities where patients see medical or administrative personnel for any kind of diagnosis, treatment, or interaction. Next, let's define the basic actors in *the system*: the *patient* is on the receiving end of some kind of medical intervention, the *provider* offers or performs the intervention, and the *payer* is responsible for the financial cost for that intervention. With that out of the way, we can lead into the details that make this all so complicated.

Who Pays, and How

Fundamentally, medical billing is about other people's money. Anything that happens to patients in *the system* is expensive—very, very expensive. We will look into why that is often the case later in this chapter, but take our word for it: if you haven't already had an outrageously high medical bill or two, you probably will. As a result of that high expense, the overwhelming majority of patients are not able to directly pay for the services they incur when they enter the system and this is where the payers step in. What might first come to mind is the traditional medical insurance company; they are definitely in the payer category. However, thousands of other organizations pay for some or all of the services for different and specialized parts of the population:

- Large companies that directly pay for medical services, acting as their own insurance company for their employees
- Workers' compensation systems that pool funds and pay for medical services in specific cases
- Government funds such as Feca/Black Lung, which pay only for treatment of a specific diagnosis
- Other government funds that are disease-specific, such as Ryan White, which pays for most care but only for HIV/AIDS patients

And there are easily thousands of other unique payers who defy categories. Finally, patients themselves are burdened with some amount of individual financial responsibility in most transactions.

Claims

Now that we have defined the large number of potential payers of all shapes and sizes, we need to discuss the fundamental transaction of medical billing: the *claim*. The claim can be thought of a bit like an invoice in other industries, with one vital difference: you almost never get the amount you ask for on the claim.

Many people might be surprised to learn that even now, a large number of medical claims are completely paper transactions from end to end. Although not terribly important to the overall workflow, we'll mention here the CMS1500 and CMS1450 physical paper forms so that you are familiar with the terms. The CMS1500, also sometimes still called the HCFA1500, is the name of the paper form used to communicate a claim for a patient who was seen in an outpatient interaction. CMS1450, or sometimes still called the UB-04, is the equivalent paper form for a patient seen in an inpatient interaction. The forms are rarely but diligently filled out in pen, more commonly printed on a laser printer, or somewhat unbelievably still printed with dot-matrix printers.

The purpose of the medical claim document, whether the paper form just mentioned or in an electronic format discussed next in this chapter, is to communicate the precise actions, tools, and supplies that were provided or used in the patient interaction with the provider. Each of those is itemized and priced. Alongside that is information about the facility, the provider, and the patient. Those details include national identification numbers, tax identifiers, specialized codes for the actions performed called procedure codes, specialized codes for the diagnoses or reasons justifying those actions, special codes for supplies, and finally itemized prices associated with each of the specialized procedure codes.

Paper forms were the standard medical claim in several different versions since the inception of Medicare in the 1960s, and as we mentioned continue to be used today in a surprisingly large number of instances. When HIPAA was passed in 1996, it attempted to standardize a new electronic format for medical billing. That format leveraged electronic data interchange technology originally invented in the 1970s known as ANSI 837. Although the format was still somewhat contemporary at the start of its adoption in the 1990s, it is terribly antiquated today, but deeply entrenched efforts to modernize again have fallen flat. So today medical billing claims exist as either very antiquated paper documents or a very antiquated electronic format.

Now that the terminology bounding the medical workflow has been discussed, we can look at the workflow in more detail.

Eligibility

The first element of medical billing occurs before the patient has actually been seen by the provider and when he or she first enters into the facility to receive services. This first step can be categorically called *eligibility* and is a determination about the patient's ability to pay for the services to be received. If the patient has insurance, several questions come into play, such as whether the information provided by the patient corresponds with the insurer's records, whether the insurance is up to date, whether the insurance will cover the provider(s) to be involved in the care, and to what financial extent the services will be covered. In emergency situations, this eligibility step does not generally occur until after treatment has begun. However, in almost all other scenarios, eligibility has a profound effect on the availability, type, means, and service level of treatment. Many medical personnel might object to this last statement, seeing it as controversial or even offensive, but in the authors' opinion based on more than 20 years of collective experience in managing medical workflows, it is incontrovertible.

The ability of patients to meet potential financial obligations dramatically affects their path through the system. The hoops that many facilities must jump through to receive remuneration from payers increases significantly in inverse correlation to the patient's generosity of insurance and ability to self-pay.

The completion of the eligibility step ends with one of three general conclusions:

- The patient seems to have the insurance coverage or personal wealth to cover the care she is likely to receive.
- The patient has most of the insurance coverage for the care she'll receive and will be personally responsible for the remainder owed.
- The patient does not have sufficient insurance coverage or personal wealth to cover the likely care.

The patient might or might not owe an installment payment before she receives care, called a copayment or copay. This payment could be a fixed fee or a percentage of likely fees paid by the patient and serves two purposes. The first is a concept serving the payers that this fee is a disincentive to receive care that is not absolutely required. There is not a lot of evidence to either support or discount this concept. The second aspect of the copay is a compromise between facilities and payers that provides the facility with some amount of cash flow before the medical claims are resolved and paid, which can often take weeks or even months. Without copays, many types of facilities would need significant additional financial reserves to function while waiting for claims to be paid.

After tendering the copayment, the patient continues on to the care workflow described in Chapter 2. We will focus on some specific parts of that workflow that relate to billing after reviewing the other two eligibility determinations a patient might fall under. If the patient has only partial insurance coverage for the care she is likely to receive, the patient has to provide some financial guarantees for the remainder of charges that might occur. This is usually done in the form of a contract between the patient and the facility. The facility will attempt to collect as much remuneration as is authorized by the patient's payers, and the remaining balance will be billed to the patient directly. Involving multiple payers to cover a single patient's potential bills, and then possibly billing the patient directly, adds significant layers of complexity to the claims process.

The third determination on eligibility, that the patient has no insurance or is otherwise unlikely to be able to cover the planned services, is also very complicated. Depending on the type of provider services needed, the facility might choose to turn the patient away, alter the type of care to fit within the confines of the available payers, or attempt to supplement the available payers with additional government, charitable, or other programs. A few types of facilities treat patients regardless of their ability to pay or have payers cover services. One notable, long-term, and successful endeavor operated by the federal government is the Federally Qualified Health Center (FQHC) and Community Health Center (CHC) program, which offers higher payments for certain Medicare-insured patients in exchange for an agreement by the facility to treat all patients regardless of their coverage or personal ability to pay.

We end this discussion with new requirements introduced by meaningful use. The guidelines require a health facility to have electronic eligibility verification available, but it does not necessarily have to be used. Many large commercial (nongovernmental) payers can conduct a computerized inquiry sending the patient's information and receiving a response that confirms the patient's participation in that program and defines coverage levels. If electronic eligibility verification is not available, the information is typically input into a payer-provided website or a telephone call is made to make the determination.

Treatment

With the eligibility determination completed, the stage is set for the patient to see the provider. Chapter 2 points out several additional clinical steps that can occur, but for the purposes of the billing workflow, we can jump to the interaction between the provider and the patient. A delicate question exists about how much a patient's eligibility determination and coverage levels affect the clinical decision-making process. We don't claim a direct relationship, but the eligibility determination generally colors the range of available treatment options and patients typically must make decisions among the treatments financially accessible to them.

This takes us to a very important question that hangs over medical billing: How much does a particular interaction or treatment cost? This seems like an obvious question to many patients, but the answer, like almost everything else in medical billing, is very complicated. We can start clarifying the question further by rephrasing it: How much is the treating facility going to bill for the codes in this particular interaction? And that is a nice segue for us to talk about the fundamental unit of medical billing, the code. These codes have been mentioned a few times in this book so far, but it is important here that we break down the particular codes of importance to medical billing. These are:

Procedure codes

These come from the Current Procedure Terminology (CPT) list, updated each year by the American Medical Association. This set of codes can be differentiated from the others we will discuss next by thinking of them as a reference for what providers *do*. CPT codes identify, in little pieces, the entire set of actions by providers for which some kind of remuneration is available. For example, the code 99214 describes an "office or other outpatient visit for the evaluation and management of an established patient, which requires at least two of these three key components: a detailed history, a detailed examination and medical decision making of moderate complexity." A visit of that type is intended to take approximately 25 minutes. The provider may perform many activities with the patient, but unless a CPT code exists for it, there is no financial remuneration available to the provider. (Famously, there is no code for answering a patient's email.) At this time there are roughly 17,000 CPT codes.

Diagnosis codes

These come from a set of codes with the name ICD-9, for International Classification of Diseases. A myriad of entities are involved with the creation and maintenance of ICD-9 (see "International Classification of Diseases

(ICD)" on page 146 for details), but medical billing makes use of an adapted set of the codes called the ICD9-CM (where the CM stands for "clinical modifications"). The ICD9-CM is maintained by the National Center for Health Statistics and the Centers for Medicare and Medicaid, both of which are part of the federal government. To understand the role of diagnosis codes, you can think of them as the why that provides justification for a particular act that the provider performed. Again, the provider can perform many acts, even those that have CPT procedure codes associated with them, but unless she also provides a sufficient "why" in the form of diagnosis codes, there will be no remuneration.

Supply, nonprovider, and drug codes

These come from the HCPCS (pronounced hick-picks) set of codes and identify specific supplies, physical goods, drugs, and a catch-all assortment of acts done by nonproviders (such as ambulance services). HCPCS stands for Healthcare Common Procedure Coding System. These codes are also maintained by the Centers for Medicare and Medicaid. The codes can be thought of as a supplement to CPT codes, and for practical purposes are used interchangeably on billing forms.

There is more information on these codes and the relationships between code sets in Chapter 10.

Now let's return to the question of what the facility charges for a particular intervention represents. That stems first from the facility's assessment of its own costs: overhead, salaries, and so on. Then they look at what other facilities in their region charge and what payers pay for that action on average. They do some cost shifting from activities that might need to be done but for which no code exists, and finally include some kind of weighted factor to cover nonpayments, underpayments, and bad debt.

Bringing the various parts together, each facility assigns a distinct price to a specific code from the CPT or HCPCS list. That table of prices or fees is commonly referred to as a *fee schedule*. For accounting purposes, a facility is required to define a base or default fee schedule, although in practice some facilities might have different fee schedules that apply to cash-only patients or other specialized circumstances. It is not legal in all jurisdictions for a facility to employ multiple fee schedules.

Yet another twist is the notion of discounted fees. Many facilities participate in a variety of payer programs or incentives that apply per-interaction or per-code discounts. The most common application of discounts is for patients who are near or below the federal poverty level. Those patients might receive a flat rate pricing model, a percentage discount, or other more complex schemes. The discounts present several complicated accounting problems, especially when combined with facilities that employ multiple fee schedules for different payers.

Returning to the provider interaction with the patient, we come upon yet another complexity in answering the "how much does it cost" question. There are many more codes than a provider can possibly know off the cuff, each of which can have a distinct price. Even keeping track of the correct code for a particular action, beyond those performed routinely, is an all but impossible feat for most people. To help organize the code selection process, facilities compile a list of their most commonly employed procedure and diagnosis codes into a document or screen commonly called a superbill. The provider pulls up the superbill, ticks off the appropriate codes, and attempts to provide additional information about acts for which no quick pick code was present. That additional information will later be consulted by the medical billing staff to try to determine codes that might be applicable, if any.

A simple visit to check out a patient's persistent cough can quickly become something much more complex due to the breath sounds found when using the stethoscope. That could lead to X-rays, blood tests, and a referral to a specialist. The prevalence of chronic diseases such as diabetes also greatly complicates care and coding such that what might be a routine visit for a relatively minor cut with stitches can veer off into treatment and diagnosis of numerous complications. Maybe the cut was caused by the patient losing balance due to poorly controlled blood sugar. Because of the layers of details in those instances it can be very difficult for a provider during the interaction to capture all of the nuances of the interaction with codes. That can be done much more deliberately by a biller reviewing the free-form notes.

If the superbill is a paper form, data entry will need to be done into the billing system at a later point. Use of an electronic system by the provider means that some review might be done by billing staff, but the data entry step can be avoided.

At the point the patient has completed treatment and is being discharged or otherwise leaving a facility, a facility typically tries to collect any balance that it is certain will not be covered by a payer.

Billing

With the encounter information in hand, the heart of the medical billing workflow really begins. The staff of the medical billing department first perform an audit to make sure they have all the records for all treatments and interactions that might have occurred. The easiest place to surrender money in a medical workflow is to lose track of services, supplies, and treatments that were provided. For paper-based facilities, this process can be particularly arduous as physical paper needs to be rounded up. For electronic systems, the process might be a little easier but there are still plenty of possibilities for misrecorded or conflicting entries.

The Billing Process

Now that all the information about what has been done reaches the billing staff, their job is to coalesce that information into medical claims. For simple interactions, when the providers were able to select mainly from the predefined pick lists, a claim can be generated pretty easily. When providers delivered nonroutine treatment, a superficial review of notes might be sufficient to identify the proper codes. However, a detailed review of the entire medical record could be needed to properly assess what is appropriate to bill on the claim.

Now is a good point to talk about billing staff in general and whether they are part of the providing organization. Two cottage industries have developed within the system to facilitate medical billing: *billing services* and *clearinghouses*.

A billing service is really an outsourced billing department that receives either the paper or the electronic data about interactions and performs the billing activities on behalf of the facility. Billing services most commonly take a percentage of claim revenue recovered as payment for services. As providers install EHRs and do more electronic claims processing from start to finish, billing services are seeing declines in business. Once you have a mostly electronic workflow, billing services are usually a poor value, because historically their value proposition has been based on the outsourcing of data entry functions in addition to claims processing.

Clearinghouses act as a go-between from the provider's billing systems to the payers' electronic claims systems. As we discussed, there are many hurdles and steps in sending electronic claims, and clearinghouses have experience addressing the more common problems that payers might introduce. Some even have very elaborate preprocessing systems that conduct their own review of claims before they reach payers and can often be set up to automatically fix certain problems before final transmittal of the claims data to the payer.

One other very popular service many clearinghouses provide is called *combined ERA*. We discuss ERA claim responses later in this chapter, but suffice it to say that combined ERAs are a lot like having a copier that collates printed copies for you. Without a combined ERA, a facility has to do a lot of manual organizing and sorting of claim payment information. Clearinghouses typically charge a flat monthly fee per provider or a flat fee for each claim they transmit. The return on investment of using a clearinghouse varies widely, and most specialize in particular medical areas, so there are no good generalizations about whether a particular clearinghouse is appropriate for a specific provider. More often than not, smaller organizations employ clearinghouses until they are large enough to command direct and favorable attention from the highest volume payers they work with.

The claims themselves are a snapshot of patient demographic details, payer information, facility information, and the coding that was done by the provider and updated by the billing staff. For each procedure code, the biller constructs a claim line that consists of, at a minimum, the procedure code, one or more justifying diagnosis codes, and the billed amount based on the facility's fee schedule. For paper claims, the information is placed onto the forms and mailed or faxed. Thankfully, paper claims are beginning to be the exception rather than the rule. Electronic claims are finalized and transmitted directly to a payer or intermediary via a modem over dial-up (still common for governmental payers) or over the Internet.

Complexities in Billing

The justification of procedures presents several challenges for practices. For each individual procedure, one or more diagnosis codes must be used to justify the procedure, taking into account the order of the diagnoses. The first listed diagnosis is considered the primary justification, with the additional ones considered supplementary. It is uncommon, but not unheard of, to use more than four diagnoses to justify a single procedure. Where the justification becomes tricky is that, in most workflows, the provider has neither the time nor inclination to make the extremely detailed and nuanced decisions that are necessary to qualify a procedure to make sure that it's expressed in a way that will be paid. Many smaller facilities think that adopting an EHR will eliminate or reduce the need for specialized billing staff (either outsourced or direct employees). Unfortunately, this is not true for several reasons, one of them being the complexity of claim justification.

When the billing staff finalizes the claim, we arrive at the first time in the workflow that there really is some indication of what the patient could potentially owe. However, that amount is only a theoretical calculation of the amount the practice will ultimately receive because of possible denial or underpayment by the provider, and because of the difficulties in recouping 100% of remaining costs from the patients or others who are financially responsible for the services that were provided.

Finalization takes many forms, but one consistent step is the application of *edits*. These are errata or addenda, based on experience or a computer system, that make small adjustments to the coding to account for peculiarities of individual payers and coding situations. The computer software can be purchased or contracted out. In some cases, edits trigger a warning on a claim. In other cases, they automatically translate coding data from the values originally entered into an altered form that will appear on the claim. Edits can save a lot of time by avoiding refusals or denials for procedural rather than clinical or contractual reasons. Medicare is the pinnacle of complexity in this regard, and an entire subagency with a staff of several hundred people is employed to produce two very large data sets that can be used in electronic edits systems and by other payers in their back-end processing.

Facilities that have been operating for a while begin to construct their own unique list of edits based on experience with claims for their unique line of care and patient population. A good feature for electronic billing systems is some type of claim rules engine (CRE) that automatically applies relevant edits to each claim that is created.

Medicare, which maintains its own comprehensive set of coding guidance, produces enormous data sets for automated computer checking that are collectively referred to as the National Correct Coding Initiative (NCCI). The NCCI consists of two very large data sets:

Mutually Exclusive Codes list
Procedure codes that cannot or should not appear on the same claim. A simple example might be the application of both the 99213 and 99214 procedure codes on a single claim. Each of those codes represents an established patient visit with different length and complexity, so there is no realistic way that both codes could be applicable on a single claim.

Medically Unlikely Edits list
Combinations that, for clinical reasons, are very unlikely to occur on the same claim and will receive the maximum level of scrutiny by the payer.

If one spins out all the combinations possible with these lists, they cover more than 2 billion (yes, billion) coding possibilities.

Just for the sake of completeness, there is also a third secret data set colloquially referred to as the Fraud Watch list. It is disseminated only within CMS and to its contractors and is protected with a large amount of secrecy. This list encompasses coding combinations that Medicare believes, or has evidence to show, are being exploited for the purposes of fraud. A facility that frequently submits claims with large numbers of hits on the fraud list is flagged for auditing by Medicare. The list is kept secret so as not to alert the fraud perpetrators and to prevent its use as a dictionary for committing fraud. Private payers have similar, if less sophisticated, systems in place.

Adjudication

Adjudication is the payer's process for resolving a claim and—if it is deemed valid—determining a payment. Usually, facilities get paid much less than the face value of the claims. Paper claims can undergo incredibly long volleys of resubmitting a claim and receiving a written response. Electronic claims generally pass through several specific adjudication steps:

1. The format of the claim is validated. The intricacy of the 837 technology leaves plenty of room for problems in formatting. An electronic claim can be refused by the receiving systems immediately on submission, or more commonly after some kind of processing delay caused by the need for parsing and format checking. These refusals have nothing to do with the merits of the claim, but simply mean that the receiving system could not digest the document. Every payer and program has subtle and distinct rules and parameters about the electronic format they will accept. Attempts by HIPAA to define a rigid, standard claim format have not unified the marketplace. Part of the difficulty is technological, because different payers employ difference processing systems with unique properties. But part of the bar-

rier is intentional, to make sending claims as cumbersome as possible. Several cottage industries have popped up to address the opaque process required simply to prevent a claim from being refused electronically by payers' systems. When a claim is refused electronically, the biller or their agent can make corrections and retransmit it, so a loop can occur as many times as necessary to get the claim's transmission accepted.

2. Once an electronic claim has been successfully transmitted, the payer's system evaluates the enclosed demographic, policy, and coding information. This could take hours or even days to complete. It is routine for claims to be denied at this point for very minor problems, including subtle mismatches of name, address, and policy information. *Denial*, which is the name for rejection at this point, is different from *refusal*, which the electronic system could generate at the previous stage. Depending on the specific reason for the denial, the facility can revise the claim and resubmit it with the correct information. This can sometimes require follow-up with the provider or patient. Claims submissions are typically limited by the payer to a set number of denials (after which they will not pay) as part of the contract between the facility and the paying organization.

3. Should a claim successfully complete validation, it is then reviewed on clinical and contractual grounds, taking into account the type of care, the patient's policy and contract with the paying organization, the facility's contracts, and so forth. Not all services a provider might deliver are covered by all payers in their arrangements with the provider. Some services might not be covered at all, or the patient might have some type of deductible amount or coverage ceiling that places the service outside the boundaries for compensation from the payer. This final review is the actual adjudication of the claim, and most often results in partial payment for some of the codes that were billed.

4. At this stage, payments are made on a procedure code by procedure code basis. For each line in the claim, the payer defines an amount of payment and gives a reason for any amount that is not being paid. The collective feedback on a particular claim is called an explanation of benefits (EOB) when it is delivered by paper. When it is returned electronically, it is more frequently called electronic remittance advice (ERA). In many cases, payers make errors with respect to adjudication and the facility or patient must then engage in an appeal or re-review process to resolve underpayments or denials of payment that might be unwarranted.

Already you can begin to see the enormous undertaking involved in getting payment for even a single claim. On average, it takes three attempts and resubmissions to have a claim adjudicated to the fullest extent that the provider or patient can achieve. We have to travel even further down the rabbit hole for patients whose services are potentially covered by multiple payers. Payers must be contacted in the correct order, and a claim that was partially covered by one payer must be recompiled to take into account payments to date and then sent on to the next payer, including the complete array of reviews and hurdles.

Having transmitted claims and received responses, denials, and adjudications, a facility will eventually receive payment for the services provided. For claims sent via paper, the timeline to actual payment can be very long, in the worst cases stretching out to almost a year from the date the services were provided to the patient. For electronic claims the timeline is significantly better most of the time, with the actual delivery of payment in 7 to 30 days.

The Patient's Burden

It might seem as though the billing workflow is close to completion with the reception of payment from the payer, but unfortunately that is far from the truth. Having received the EOB or ERA, a facility must reconcile the information provided with the balances they billed out on the claim and figure out the patient's responsibility for any remaining amount owed. Once payment is received from one payer, a claim might then need additional rebilling to one or even two more payers. After exhausting third-party payers, the billing staff must then begin a patient billing process, sending out statements and following up with patients to receive final remuneration on the services that were provided. There is no end to the complexity here. For instance, patients who are billed about a remaining balance might choose to engage in appeals and processes for resolution with their responsible payers.

The final statistics on dollars in and dollars out are pretty grim for healthcare facilities. It is uncommon that they receive more than 85 cents from payers for each dollar billed on claims and another 5 cents from patients for the remaining amount owed. Some specialties fare much better than average, whereas some specialties and particularly general practice medicine tend to fare worse.

The steps by which a billing staff follows up with patients and payers in collecting amounts owed is not all that different from those steps performed by any business that collects money for services already delivered, simply the handling of accounts receivable. The involvement of third-party payers certainly makes it more difficult in the healthcare system, along with the life impacts of medical treatment. Treatment can represent the most stressful time for people and families, and they could perceive the activities to collect money that might be owed as insult on top of literal injury.

The long potential delay between when an interaction occurs and when a facility might receive payments from a payer can also present a further hurdle for the facility ultimately collecting a balance from the patient. Many months after the fact, patients might have forgotten the details of the interaction, failed to budget for the charges, or had other significant life changes including moving jobs and insurance, or just plain moving. Dollars outstanding to patients typically take at least 30 days and as long as 18 months to collect. At that point, the bills are either sent to a collection agency or forgone as irrecoverable debt.

In concluding this discussion about medical billing, it is worthwhile to ignore the sometimes overwhelming complexity of it and to take away the crucial elements, which are these:

- The concept of "other people's money" and the hurdles that this introduces
- The inability to make broad generalizations because of the diversity of scenarios
- The magnitude of work it takes to get any payment at all in healthcare versus other industries

CHAPTER 4

The Bandwidth of Paper

When considering what an EHR could and should be, we must carefully admit that a custom paper-form-based record system is awfully hard to beat, from the perspective of the doctor that designed it. It can be as comprehensive as the user needs, and it can be modified and extended at any time by modifying the form template or by making diagrams on a specific patients form. With the judicious use of check boxes a form becomes blazingly fast, but the check boxes are not traps; each check box supports infinite extensibility. Paper degrades very slowly, and we have paper medical records that date back at least a century. Fast, durable, extensible, intuitive, convenient, forgiving, and cheap. We have not even mentioned post-it notes.

Consider the partial form in Figure 4-1.[1]

In the "history" section of the form, which is obviously very complex, the nurse had written "Polimyer Ciders" after the patient had told her that she had "polymyositis." Sounds like a mistake, right? This is funny, which is why it was posted on the Internet. Being funny does not keep this example from showing just how smart the paper process is. The nurse had written the phrase with a question mark. She had known that she did not understand what the patient was talking about, but passed along what she had heard, along with her confusion about it. Notice that "HTN," which stands for hypertension, is also checked. There is space here for a person to make notes, as the nurse did, but still clearly mark with a simple "x" the most common healthcare issues faced by typical patients. Diabetes, hypertension, heart disease, stroke, asthma, high cholesterol, and cancer are all options here. Note the expectant colon ':' in the cancer check box, calling for whoever is writing to record what type of cancer the patient had, if they chose to use the cancer check box. Paper is flexible enough to cover the strange stuff, yet fast on typical tasks.

Consider the blank sheet of plain white paper. A sheet of paper can become legal notes for a lawyer, the design of a machine or circuit for an engineer, the careful drawing of

---

1. Photo   (*http://www.flickr.com/photos/iphonepics/2097983731/sizes/m/in/photostream/*)   taken   by 'iphoneuser' on Flickr, and republished under a Creative Commons license.

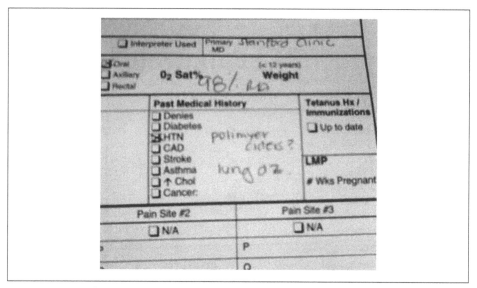

Figure 4-1. Paper form

a building for an architect, and notes about a patient for a doctor. When you account for paper airplanes and origami, paper has a wonderfully large number of wonderful uses.

The powerful aspect of a paper chart is that there is never a limitation of the type or content of data that can be added. If it can be written or drawn, it can be added as needed.

The recently released Apple Retina display is 326 pixels per inch (PPI), and normal humans cannot see clearly past 300 PPI. In the HDMI video standard, monitors must support 30-bit color on the low end. An 8-1/2 x 11-inch sheet of paper comes out to 8,415,000 pixels at 300 DPI (more HD than the most uber-HD monitors now available). Assuming they support a 30-bit color depth, this means that they are supporting 252,450,000 bits per image, or about 31 MB per image. Of course, the human eye is capable of seeing many of these pages per second, but the real limitation of the paper system is a human's ability to change sheets of paper quickly. Assuming the doctor was really moving, he might see 5 pages per second. That puts the bandwidth of paper at something like 1262.25 megabits per second (Mbps). In comparison, a good broadband Internet connection runs at about 5 Mbps, which is enough to stream movies. If you account for the fact that a doctor might be dynamically ignoring 995 pages of medical record to look at the right 5 pages, and then considered her rate of consumption at 1,000 pages per second, the bandwidth of paper is faster, by far, than any computer network in practical existence. All of these numbers are estimates, but it would be difficult for anyone not to concede that the actual bandwidth of paper-to-brain is pretty fast.

Moreover, it is easy to make paper better at any given information task. It is simple for any doctor to use a computer or photocopier to print lines and labels all over the blank sheet of paper, turning a simple sheet of paper into a form. Paper forms in healthcare are far more potent than in most industries.

When doctors look at a paper form, they feel no loyalty to the lines and check boxes. Doctors are not mere paper pushers or automatons who fill in everything in triplicate. Doctors feel comfortable drawing "outside the lines" and because they often create their own forms, and are frequently the only readers of their own completed forms, the paper-based patient data system melds easily with the mind of the designing physician. This is all just the benefits of a single paper form; when you add a folder to keep groups of forms together, it becomes even more powerful.

Instructions, diagrams, complaints, compliments, questions, answers, tables, pictures, reports, receipts, faxes, and, of course, post-it notes can all be added to a paper chart, normally just a folder, with ease. Doctors' handwriting is famously illegible, but they rarely need to actually read the entire contents of a chart. They need to be able to use the written record of what they wrote to jog their memory: what is special or different about this patient, what are the next steps in the treatment? During typical operations the chart need only indicate what the next step is to the doctor who made it. But it is still powerful enough to hold the entire history (assuming the handwriting problem is addressed), for the rare occasions when it is important to look at everything.

The nurse who filled out the example form in Figure 4-1 also wrote "Lung DZ" in the history section. That phrase means "Lung Disease," and is a wonderful example of medical abbreviations, an important part of the paper chart that will make the jump to electronic charts. Medical abbreviations are now largely standardized, after a substantial number of medical errors occurred because of nonstandard abbreviations. The standardization of abbreviations bounds written data, even on paper forms. Once medical abbreviations became standardized, they provided a clear enough shorthand for common medical terms that they could safely be recommended for use. But this is only possible when the mapping between abbreviations and longer terms is perfectly understood and mostly identical everywhere. That mapping, between abbreviations and longer terms, is in fact a healthcare ontology, one that performs well on paper. We will discuss medical abbreviations further in Chapter 10.

Workflow Tokens

Individual paper forms are typically tokens in a complex clinical workflow. The nurse fills out a form when the patient arrives and gives the patient a copy. The patient then takes it to the X-ray department. The X-ray department performs an X-ray and gives the results (on paper and film) to the patient to take upstairs to a particular doctor. The nurse in the waiting room takes the papers and film, and deposits them in a wall-mounted box outside an exam room, and escorts the patient into the room. Each of the steps can have a check box on the form itself, so that the patient knows just where to go next, and if she gets lost (and who doesn't in a hospital?) anyone can look at the form and show the patient where to go next. There are thousands of variations on this basic theme to accommodate the various needs of different clinical organizations.

This is an important insight that merits highlighting: even the paper chart (i.e., the whole bundle, not just a single form) is not just a paper record of a patient's healthcare history and current status. It is also a token in a clinical workflow. Considering the record without considering the workflow is a simple mistake that is easy for technologists to repeatedly make. To prevent this mental error, try to adjust your mental imagery of a paper chart into something dynamic and moveable in nature. One of the authors tries to imagine the record as a manila folder with little wheels attached to it. That is a pretty silly mnemonic, but it works.

Some clinics use colored folders to enable different workflows. They place the chart in a green folder and send the patient to the green waiting room. A red folder might mean that a patient is waiting in the red waiting room, and in another clinic it might mean that a patient needs to have blood drawn. As we say elsewhere, there is no such thing as a typical healthcare workflow. At a minimum the paper chart is the home base to the various paper forms that enable different clinical workflows, and the whole contents must be copied to other organizations or departments when the patient moves. So the paper chart is always a workflow token, exercised to different degrees, in different organizations.

Often, a paper form will have been designed and cemented in the workflow so long ago that no current employee can remember why the form was designed in a particular way. Be very careful of this, because as you seek to replace the form in the workflow with software, you might discover that what you considered an incidental aspect of the form's design was actually solving some important problem in another portion of the workflow that you did not fully understand.

Why Leave Paper?

Paper is an excellent record of clinical care, to the degree that the data does not need to move. It is a perfect healthcare record to the degree that healthcare is provided by a single clinician, looking at a patient chart and the patient all at the same time. Modern healthcare is no longer a one-doctor, one-record, one-patient game. The coordination of care for a patient requires that critical information be moved from where it is to where it needs to be, on time. Sometimes the paper chart moves fast enough. Most of the time it does not. God forbid a paper chart should be lost.

The first thing that people assume when you say "coordination of care" is that you mean between-organization coordination. But the primary benefit of EHR systems is that they coordinate care within a healthcare organization. This is why EHR adoption has been so strongly correlated with the size of a clinical organization. The more an organization needs to communicate with itself about a given patient, the greater the benefit of an EHR system. Conversely, single-clinician practices get the least benefit from computerization.

There are classes of medical errors that are clearly related to the information not moving fast enough, like a patient's allergies or current medication list not being with the nurse when a new drug is given to a patient. Many preventable medical errors go away entirely when you measure them, which means they mostly disappear whenever manual observation occurs. The spread of infections due to clinicians forgetting to wash their hands is a good example of this. The only real solution is to measure these types of behaviors all the time electronically, preferably preventing rather than merely chronicling the errors in question. Real-time workflow interruption can only occur when data values can spawn real-world stimuli (like flashing lights or beeps), and that means software.

Lastly, paper charts are difficult to study en masse. Doctors can easily look at a single paper chart and see how a patient with diabetes is doing, but they cannot get the same information about all of their patients with diabetes without doing costly and slow chart reviews. Paper chart reviews simply cannot serve to inform a profession that changes as fast as healthcare does.

Paper data is trapped, inactive, and difficult to study. If paper could shout, there would be no need for EHR systems.

Step 0: Health IT Humility

The first thing that computer technologists must free themselves from is the notion that computers are the "solution" to information flow in a clinical environment. If computer specialists do not understand everything that a paper process is doing, or fail to respect the ways in which a paper-based information system handles something well, then they will appear arrogant to the clinical staff, who understand perfectly how effective the paper forms can be. When you introduce a computer system that makes a process that used to take 30 seconds take 10 minutes, then your solution will instantly be met with derision by clinical staff who are already overworked.

If you want a concrete example of how good paper is, consider the surgical checklist movement that has been growing in popularity. Studies have shown that this simple information intervention, which uses either a paper form or a whiteboard, has improved patient safety on the operating table more than any surgical technique advancement in the equivalent time frame. The next time you are feeling smug about your awesome health IT plans, keep in mind that this simple information intervention, which required no software at all, might be the most effective information-based intervention of the decade.

Clinical staff, especially nurses, are well-practiced in silent rebellion against unreasonable directions by a multitude of "pointy-haired" bosses, especially when those directions interfere with their care of patients. In their hearts, the clinical staff will plot against the new software, waiting patiently until the computer trainer has left, and then use any excuse to revert to a paper workflow. Months later, a review of the software deployment will reveal that the system had been abandoned for months, despite the project being regarded as a success by management. Countless deployments of health IT software have failed because of this type of rebellion. This problem is so prevalent that you should assume healthcare staff have always reverted back to a paper process, until random spot checks have proved otherwise for months. If possible the real-time usage data (but never the contents) of an EHR system should be an item that an organization monitors within its network operations center (or equivalent). At a minimum, usage data should be logged in a way that can be studied later. Do not assume that you understand how your health IT system is being used: know.

The first step in combating user abandonment is to be realistic and humble about the benefits of any health IT system in comparison to a paper system. This cannot happen without fully respecting how really brilliant paper forms can be in healthcare workflow. Being arrogant is the first rookie mistake in deploying health IT software.

The second rookie mistake in deploying health IT systems is to attempt to replicate the patient chart in software. Ironically, this mistake comes from giving too much respect to the paper form. This is a frequent mistake made by computer programmers and purchasers who come to recognize the complexities of an effective paper-based workflow. They make the reasonable assumption that if they perfectly replicate a paper form in the health IT software, then they cannot fail to successfully replicate the nuances of that workflow.

Sadly, although that is a *reasonable* assumption, it is utterly incorrect. Almost all early attempts to computerize clinical workflows began life as an attempts to clone a patient chart in software. Many mature computer software systems still maintain some paper chart analogies, while abandoning any real parallels to paper-like designs. In fact you can reasonably assume that to the degree an EHR system actually works identically to a paper chart, it is an immature design.

Software and paper are both amazingly capable information systems. They just happen to be very good at different types of information tasks. A computer program that directly imitates a paper-based clinical workflow is doomed to be worse than both the original paper process and an effective health IT software deployment. It is usually simple to determine when this is happening. Paper-based workflows are advanced, but they are not perfect. Computers can make most things that required lengthy workflows instantaneous. When you accelerate a paper-based workflow 1,000 times, small flaws in the fundamental paper workflow become 1,000 times worse. This is why health IT advocates must understand the "why" of paper forms as much as the static health data in question. If you are adding data fields to an EHR system from a preexisting paper form without understanding the role of those data fields in the paper workflow, you will regret it.

A good rule of thumb is that a technologist should be given a five-minute lecture on any given clinical data point and its role in the clinical workflow, until the technologist is comfortable actually giving such a brief lecture themselves. This is not a paragraph to just skip over. This is the heart of the technologist plus clinician collaboration that has made the most successful clinical software deployments work. If this is not happening constantly, as a natural part of your deployment or development process, then it needs to be formalized into a ongoing process. If you have trouble formalizing this process, read up on pair programming or agile software development and consider using some of those methods with clinician-technologist pairs. Unless a technologist has a reliable, if superficial, understanding of the clinical processes in a given clinical environment, the technology deployment will be misdirected. This level of familiarity takes time and is expensive. Be suspicious of any technologist who underestimates this expense, especially if he or she is not very familiar with health IT.

Do not think this advice does not apply to you if you are not actually conducting software development on the core of an EHR. When you deploy an EHR system, you are developing software. Your chosen EHR is simply your programming substrate. If you are thinking of your deployment of an EHR as a minor software development effort you will be better prepared for the level of engineering you will need to do in order to replace a paper-based data and workflow system.

Paper handles ambiguity extremely well. Remember the nurse who filled in the check box with a question mark? She was dynamically repurposing the paper form to communicate a complex ambiguity. With a software check box widget, which must be either checked or unchecked, there is no option for "repurposed." Imagine the conundrum that this creates for the EHR software developer/deployer. To fully account for the case where a midlevel clinical professional, like a nurse, is unsure about a detail of the patient's history, the software developer must force the nurse to make a choice that she in unsure of (she does not really know whether she should "check" or not), to somehow record the fact that she was uncomfortable somehow, and then find a way for the higher-level provider to override that clinical decision in an elegant way. That is a lot of software intelligence to replace something that the paper form does intrinsically.

If you want to replace a paper chart or even migrate from a previous software-based system, you must fully understand what the old and new systems are capable of. Elegant and advanced health IT software has different ways of dealing with healthcare workflows. The most useful tool in your effort to "develop" your EHR system is to understand the two basic approaches to recording health data: liberally formatted input and usefully bounded input.

Normalized Data

Just because you are storing data does not mean that you are storing it well. Certain data storing software (relational databases) have a concept called *normalization*. For now, we can skip an exact definition of what relational databases are and what, precisely, normalization means in that context. Those of you who are already familiar with normalization (as it applies to databases, not statistics) will quickly be comfortable with our use of this term. For our purposes, we will use the term normalization to mean data that is:

Well bounded
> The potential values in the data are usefully constrained.

Well linked
> The relationships between different data points are well understood.

Flexible
> Carefully violating the first two rules only when required to do something faster, better, or differently.

If the patient data in an EHR is well bounded and well linked, it is easy to leverage for higher level processes like reporting, clinical decision support, data exchange, and other useful clinical automations. The simplest useful function that an EHR can perform with normalized data is accurate and comprehensive reporting. The basic function that underlies data reporting is data grouping, which in healthcare means grouping patients based on some data about them. The meaningful use standards require smoking status reporting, for instance, and that is only possible with normalized smoking data.

Normalized data allows you to ask questions of your patients as a population. In some ways, the term *electronic* in electronic health record is ironic. Merely storing patient data on computers does not, by itself, allow a patient population to be studied more effectively. There are at least two examples of health IT approaches that certainly count as electronic, but do not qualify as an EHR as per meaningful use. The first is simply a collection of word processing documents. Many physician power users created methods of very effectively creating piles and piles of text documents about their patients. Although these power users benefited greatly from their automations, this did not create data in a way that would allow grouping. Similarly, many in the health IT industry have historically maintained that the purpose of computer systems should be to merely archive and organize scans of paper charts. The meaningful use standards made it clear that these approaches were unacceptable. Of course, both of these approaches could be part of a system that qualified as an EHR under meaningful use, but they do not qualify without software that meets requirements that are impossible without structured data.

Information exchange between clinical sites is impossible to automate without normalized data. For information exchange to take place, data must not only be normalized (i.e., well-structured), but it must be structured in a specific way. One of the tasks that is relatively simple for computers to execute is the conversion of one form of structured data to another. Different forms of structured data have different benefits. Specific data structure formats allow the transfer of clinical data from one party to another and we will discuss those in detail in Chapter 11. For now it is important to emphasize that without well-structured clinical data as a starting point, it is impossible to generate data in a structure that can facilitate the exchange of clinical information. This means there is no point in moving to an EHR system without normalized data because without adequate structure, there is no way for computerized patient data to coordinate care better than paper records.

Other resources, including the meaningful use standards, refer to normalized data as "structured data" but that ignores the possibility that the structure is wrong. Normalized, for our purposes, means well-structured and working. Not all structure is created equal. Substantial portions of this book will be spent discussing what well-structured data looks like.

If EHR software is not providing well-bounded and well-linked data, it is really no better, and often much worse, than paper charts. The important thing for clinicians to understand is that the data must be linked and bounded correctly. That might seem obvious to a technologist. What the technologist needs to understand is that linking and bounding clinical data is a complex clinical decision. Clinicians often defer this complicated medical issue by designing paper forms, with boundaries that are easy to repurpose on a case-by-case basis.

Good Boundaries Mean Good Data

The paper form check box and the software check box only seem similar. The paper version can be marked with a question mark, in the case of a confused clinical staff member. It can be the source of an arrow drawn to a note written elsewhere in on the form. In short it can, and often does, all kinds of information tasks. Obviously a paper form check box can also be checked or not checked.

The check box element of standard graphical user interfaces (GUIs; the part of software that you actually see on the screen), can only do one of those tasks. It can be on. It can be off. In fact, the check box can represent any two arbitrary states: hungry or not hungry, etc.

The advantage of the software check box is that it is strongly bounded. By limiting the choices to only two possibilities it forces the clinical user to place the patient into one of two categories. Once a patient has been categorized in this way, it is possible for the software to leverage this in countless automated tasks. Most of the meaningful use standards are focused on the contents of the reports that a mature EHR system can generate, and without well-bounded data these reports are impossible. Let's look at two examples of how a check box can be used or abused in clinical software.

The first simple example is the test for HIV status. The HIV lab test can actually have more than just positive and negative results, but results are typically retested until a person can be considered clearly either HIV positive or negative. Using a simple check box, a user can mark a patient as HIV positive. That allows the software to include other information about the patient's health in reports for all the patients that are HIV positive. Forcing a distinction between HIV positive and negative and excluding the ambiguities involved in the test is a useful thing to do. It allows the software to provide warnings to clinical users to protect themselves from HIV infection using double latex gloves when appropriate. There are countless other clinical workflows that change based on HIV status. Using a software check box to force a clinician into making a yes or no decision makes the software more capable of clinically useful tasks.

Many technologists are used to similarly exclusive options (usually using exclusive radio buttons, which is another type of software GUI element) for male or female. In fact, this is the perfect example of the type of two-value choices that are appropriate in typical software design (like accounting software or web-based store fronts), but totally inappropriate for clinical software. For any clinician there are at least three genders: male, female, and other (as in "You better pay attention to this clinical issue"). For any clinician who treats gender-related conditions there are many, many more. It is clinically dangerous to ignore gender-related clinical issues by forcing clinicians to choose either male or female.

HIV status can be usefully bounded as a yes or no question, but gender cannot be bounded as just XX or XY. On a paper form, "male" and "female" are safe options because you can clearly mark any third choice in countless ways. Gender designation is a controversial and subtle health information issue, and a good example for the difficult requirements for health software. Health software has to get a thousand subtle data bounding issues right just to be on par with paper. Checking to see how many options are available for gender is a great way to determine how mature an EHR system is. If there are only two choices, the software should be considered dangerously immature.

Bounding also has another general principle: have only one copy of a given data in the database. Once you consider the difficulties of having two or more copies, the reason for this quickly becomes apparent. Let's suppose we have HIV status recorded in two places in the database: place A and place B. Normally this happens when two different subsystems in an EHR need to leverage the same piece of data. We can imagine that place A is in the surgical planning portion of the EHR and place B is the HIV status on the main patient chart.

Obviously, knowing whether a patient has HIV before a surgery is critically important. It makes sense to make an extra HIV question part of the presurgery workflow. The workflow is implicitly asking the patient: "Hey, last week when we scheduled this surgery, we asked you if you were HIV positive and you said no...but I am giving you one more chance to answer that question differently..." and then explicitly: "Are you HIV positive?" usually on a presurgery form. The workflow pretty much has to be this way. Sometimes people are reluctant to share important health information, and the workflow has to give people multiple opportunities to share this information.

But just because the workflow has to ask the question twice does not mean that the information system should have two places in the database where the information can exist. Let's continue to imagine that the presurgery HIV status has its own place in the database. Obviously, the whole reason that the second HIV question exists in the workflow is because, occasionally, a patient will answer "Yes" to the question only immediately before the surgery. Sometimes, the value of the first HIV status will be "No" and the presurgery HIV status will be "Yes." It is also possible to have the main HIV status be "Yes" and the presurgery HIV status be "No," but usually this is a data entry error.

So what do "Yes/No" or "No/Yes" items mean? Obviously, these data items have no reliable meaning. They must be reconciled. The need for reconciliation is common when you have two separate software systems, and we will talk more about how to deal with these type of issues in Chapter 11. But it should never happen within the same information system. Normalization requires that a single piece of data occur only one time in a given information system. If you find that there are two places to record an identical piece of data in a particular system, that is evidence of a flawed design.

That brings us to this rule: Have only one copy of any given piece of data. Instead of copying data into two places on the system, instead link data from one part of the information system to the other.

Data at Peace with Itself: Linked Data

Data linking is a far more subtle and difficult issue. Data linking is all about the way data in one part of a patient's record relates to data in another part of the record. When data linking fails, the data in an EHR for a patient is at war with itself. The simplest way to ensure that data is well-linked is to try and ensure that data is always linked correctly, rather than duplicated.

Returning to gender as an example, when a new patient, Jane Doe arrives at the office, the front desk personnel was distracted and marked Jane as a "male." Later, Jane becomes pregnant. In different parts of the EHR system, the fact of Jane's pregnancy and details about her pregnancy are stored. We might wish that an EHR could warn us of such a typo, but to do this, pregnancy status must somehow be linked with gender in a way that allows the software to know that something is amiss. If a patient marked as a male has pregnancy data, the patient's record is probably at war with itself. Either linking has not occurred, or the software is not properly leveraging the links. We know that normalization requires that a single fact appear in only one place in the database. That rule is being violated here. In the pregnancy data section, the fact that the patient is female is either assumed or explicitly recorded, but it is contradicted elsewhere in the record.

It should be clear that the first two principles of normalization are really two parts of the same principle. Instead of duplicating data with the same meaning in an EHR, only one copy should be kept. Linking allows that single copy to do the work of two copies.

Flexible Data

As with many things in health IT, the exception proves the rule. Although a single copy of any given data point is always preferable, this is impossible in any EHR system that has even rudimentary interoperation with other information systems (e.g., the insurance companies' IT infrastructure). Often several copies and variations must be maintained about a data element in order to account for the differences between systems. The simplest example is when a given patient has one name that he or she prefers to use at the clinic, and another name that must be used to bill insurance.

Rather than a violation of our core concept, that data should not be replicated, we should more carefully define what a "piece" of data means. Every "First Name" field in an information system is usually not equivalent at all; rather, each copy is really a different piece of data. For instance you might have the following legitimate examples of secondary "First Name" fields.

> First Name for billing
> First Name in the name history
> First Name as recently imported from the Lab Information System (LIS)

These are all cases where you must seemingly violate the single copy rule, but by defining the fields more carefully you can see that they are not actually the identical data at all; instead, they are merely strongly related data fields.

Essentially, this allows us to again extend the "have only one copy" rule:

> Have only one copy of any given piece of data, unless you have a good reason not to. Instead, use linking to make a single data element work in different parts of a system. When this is possible, it is usually because two copies of the data have different meanings. When you have two copies, make sure to clearly differentiate why the second copy must exist. Never, under any circumstances, continually maintain two copies of the same data with identical clinical purposes.

It is acceptable for you to import a health record from another provider that has an HIV status that is opposite the one that you have for a particular patient. It is acceptable for you to maintain a different name for a patient, so that you can get billing to work. It is not acceptable, not even a little bit, for you to have two different copies for HIV status that you must rely on in different clinical situations. If your EHR system continually places you in a position where clinicians are wondering which value is correct, that is a design flaw. Mature EHR systems will not do this to clinical users.

There are cases where healthcare data is necessarily at war with itself. You must do everything you can not to add to that problem.

Assume Health Data Changes

First names, last names, eye color, and gender are all things that normal IT regards as stationary and static aspects of a person. But in fact, all of these things change in some people some of the time. Normal IT systems might allow users to update and change these "static" personal information data points, but EHR systems must allow these changes to occur and also track them over time. This is a another good indicator of mature EHR systems. If there is no mechanism for accessing the history of name changes for an individual, then you should regard the EHR as dangerously immature.

Free Text Data

The problem with trying to normalize healthcare data is that there are too many exceptions. Most patients will always have something about them that is outside the bounds of what an EHR might normally expect. The solution is simple: free text, which usually lives in a part of the record called patient notes.

Free text has many of the same benefits of paper. With enough text, almost any subtlety can be made clear. Free text has no bounds. Like paper, it can contain whatever it needs to. Like paper, free text data has substantial limitations when compared to normalized data. When we say free text, we really just mean text, with an emphasis on the fact that one can always write anything in text GUI fields. Although it is possible for software to analyze free text information, it is unwise to rely on the results of those analysis for clinical decisions.

Imagine that the free text portion of a clinical record contains the following text:

> This *patient has had HIV* tests for many years, but they have always returned negative.

Now consider this second record:

> This *patient has had HIV* for many years, and is only now medicating properly.

In both phrases, an identical string of words appear, but in context, one person is HIV positive, and the other is not. Software can easily search all of the patient records for the phrase "has had HIV" or "has HIV" and assume that all of the patients with this text written somewhere in their EHR record are HIV positive. Of course, for some small portion of the patients, the ones with tricky text as in this example, that conclusion would be wrong. For software to be able to process free text information, it would need to be able to read, with context, as well as a human. The software would need to understand sarcasm and irony. This is a difficult task indeed, as not every human can easily parse sarcasm or irony.

Computers are very good at processing discrete data. Computers can process free text as discrete data, and come to valuable conclusions. Those conclusions cannot be relied on for life or death decisions, though. Any information that must be relied on for critical health decisions must be recorded as normalized data.

You cannot get normalized data from free text. Happily it is relatively simple to have normalized data generate free text. Many modern EHR systems allow users to first create normalized patient data, and then automatically generate free text from that data. Automatic text generation saves time and contributes greatly to the readability of the patient chart. The mechanism is simple: a doctor or nurse uses a GUI to record health information, like a check box to record HIV status, and then the software imports that data automatically into the note using automatically generated prose. In the HIV example, the software might add the sentence "The patient is HIV positive" to the note, when the check box is checked. A doctor can extend this text in meaningful ways, adding richness while saving time. He or she might write, "The patient is HIV positive, but is not yet experiencing symptoms." The small time savings gained from not needing to type the first half of this longer sentence adds up in the constantly time-constrained healthcare industry.

There are two obvious important dangers with auto-generated free text data. Both of them have to do with protecting the integrity of the normalized data.

Some systems, which have claimed falsely to be EHR systems, do not record normalized data from their GUI elements, instead electing to use the free text note as the only place the data is stored. A good example is any system that uses word processor macros to generate text documents quickly. This type of software has GUIs that could be used to save normalized data, but instead of saving the values into a database that can be normalized, it saves it only as a text document. This is a software design flaw, and cannot meet the meaningful use requirements. By definition, a system like this is not an EHR.

Some EHR users will modify the free text data to contradict the normalized data, without also modifying the normalized data. This is a user process flaw that cannot easily be corrected in software. Because free text is flexible enough to support any content there is no simple way to ensure that it does not contradict normalized data.

Now we have the background to look at a simple statement taken directly from the meaningful use standards:

> The Stage 1 meaningful use criteria, consistent with other provisions of Medicare and Medicaid law, focuses on electronically capturing health information in a structured format; using that information to track key clinical conditions and communicating that information for care coordination purposes (whether that information is structured or unstructured, but in structured format whenever feasible);

The meaningful use standards use the term structured, whereas we say normalized only to emphasize that structure is not a simple issue and must be handled carefully. Still this language demonstrates that the Department of Health and Human Services (HHS) recognizes that the distinction and capabilities inherent in free text versus structured (hopefully normalized) data are important issues. Now you should understand why.

The lesson of this chapter is simple. For the clinician it is to recognize the value of normalized or structured data. For the technologist it is to recognize that structuring of EHR data is a clinical issue. Healthcare ontologies represent the practice of bounding healthcare data. Sometimes health ontology is a science, and at other times it is a power struggle or political maneuvering. For now it is enough to say that how to bound healthcare data is best left to specialists. If you find yourself trying to imagine all of the alternatives to "male" and "female" or answering some other fundamentally clinical data bounding question, you are probably in trouble. This chapter is all about why data needs to be normalized, and Chapter 5 details how that should occur.

Herding Cats: Healthcare Management and Business Office Operations

Medical operations are often divided into administrative and clinical operations. Here we take a look at some of the key aspects of administrative activities, with an eye toward where, why, and how IT fits in. After reading this chapter, you should know where your software fits into the basic system architecture, and therefore be more likely to avoid an implementation plan that overpromises and underdelivers.

Nearly all healthcare settings have a front office that has a medical director and handles all clinical aspects of the work, and a back office under a business manager that does administration, billing, and other business functions. This has proven to be a very unfortunate division, bringing to mind a Solomonic "solution" without the happy ending. In today's world, the cost and profitability of both facilities and payers have an enormous influence on care, so the inefficiency created by the front office/back office division holds back creative efficiencies and adds significantly to the total cost for everything.

Perhaps in some earlier period there was a well-intentioned purpose to this division, such as to prevent cost and profitability concerns from having an undue impact on care. But the universal division of responsibilities is now a barrier. For instance, these two divisions often use two different software solutions provided by two different vendors, integrated by a third vendor. And meaningful use did not attempt to address the problem.

We have discussed at length the significant parts of the clinical workflow and touched on a few pieces of the healthcare management workflow, but what exactly makes up healthcare management? At a healthcare facility, it's a lot like every other business, with human resources, payroll, marketing and advertising, vendor relations, physical plant maintenance, general accounting (general ledger), and so forth.

Most facilities have employed some form of electronic healthcare management for years or even decades, but have not had an EHR system. Meaningful use puts pressure on them to adopt electronic clinical systems, but without a much thought of how they will interact with existing healthcare management systems. This presents a very counter-productive formula for continuing inefficiency and high costs.

Healthcare management can be considered the glue that holds together a healthcare organization, linking real-world financial and legal obligations with the clinical world's focus on patients and their care. Medical billing, which we covered in Chapter 3, is for the most part the only substantial bridge between both functions.

The stickiest part of healthcare management is scheduling. Second only to medical billing, medical scheduling presents enormous challenges, particularly to the traditional split between clinical and administrative functions. The scheduling of provider time touches on human resources, but certainly also has impacts on clinical operations. The scheduling of patients has a very dramatic role in clinical operations and patient care, but is also directly tied to human resources and physical plant.

In most facilities that have been in business more than a few years, patient needs outstrip resources, including persons, space, and equipment. Now we get to the most frequently asked question about healthcare and facilities: why is the doctor always running late? The answer is actually pretty simple: lack of healthcare resources. Compounding this, need and availability are very unevenly distributed across urban and rural areas and other geographic distinctions.

Unlike many large, high-volume businesses, healthcare facilities do not typically employ logistics analysis and management systems to regulate staffing and scheduling. That lack of analysis results in somewhat awkward and clunky retail hours at many types of organizations.

Appointment length is typically a function of clinical complexity, so a logistics engine would have to understand which patients are sickest. There is one simple logistics tool that is regularly applied in outpatient facilities to flexibly address the "time" problem: overbooking. Overbooking, or double-booking, is just what it sounds like—you schedule two patients for the same time slot. In theory, overbooking is a wonderful idea. If you have two patients who should take only 10 minutes each, you schedule them both for the same 30 minute block during the day. Generally, the patient who arrives first gets the first half of the overbooked slot. If both patients are clinically simple and only take up their 10 minutes, the provider ends up with a 10 minute break before the next block of overbooked patients. If one patient is twice as complex as was expected, the provider is still ready for the next block of patients on schedule. Of course, when both patients go over, the provider is late for the next block of patients. In that case, it is hoped that the next patients will be simple and the time can be recovered. All too often, several patients go long at the beginning of the day and all of the patients that follow have to wait.

Given that many schedulers have some clinical experience and are at least somewhat aware of the clinical complexity associated with particular patients, the overbooking method is often very effective. With that scheduling expertise in place, overbooking helps to ensure that the provider is always busy, but that patients do not wait too long. Some organizations extend the idea further and attempt "triple-booking". Most decent scheduling modules within EHR/practice management systems support overbooking —and in many cases, it is not concern for HIPAA compliance that prompts the shift from other scheduling systems, but the desire to support overbooking.

In fact, you could think of group therapy sessions in mental or physical therapy as a kind of nth degree overbooking. You bring lots of patients together with one provider in order to have them help heal each other. This type of optimization is pretty difficult to effectively manage with a scheduling system like Microsoft Outlook/Exchange Calendar or Google Calendar, although many many practices start there. (Yes, we know those systems are not HIPAA-compliant.)

An advanced scheduling engine in an EHR should support constraints for different combinations of appointment type, provider capacity, and patient needs. For instance, a common requirement is to ensure that all appointments for patients that speak a certain language all occur on the same day of the week: the day that the translator is also scheduled. A particular provider might decide that they want to do all non-emergent surgical pre-meetings on Mondays. An advanced scheduling module in an EHR or practice management system allows an organization to coordinate schedules to a much greater degree. Smaller organizations often prefer to have manual systems for coordinating different scheduling constraints. Often when an organization grows, these manual processes (usually reliant on a single well-informed employee) begin to break down.

Patients also bear a large responsibility for delays, particularly at outpatient facilities. They often fail to appear (no shows) or appear very late for appointments. This causes a delay like backed up trains throughout a day. Although each delay might be small, the delays are cumulative. By the afternoon, there can easily be a delay of a full interaction length or more. Although this discussion might seem like a tangent, it sets the stage for looking at what role healthcare management has in an organization.

Major Business Office Activities

In the following sections we'll take a look at the key administrative responsibilities that healthcare organizations face. If you never before appreciated the challenges and pressures faced by the support staff you have seen rushing around the clinics or hospitals you visit, you might wish to thank and sympathize with them after reading this chapter.

Insurance

If there is one time-consuming activity that dominates healthcare management, it is the follow-up, correction, and contracting of insurance relationships for patients. Patients tend to be very inconsistent sources of information concerning their own personal details, providing different details to the payer when signing up for policies and to the provider at the point of contact. Furthermore, many patients are covered only through the policies of their spouses or other relatives, and routinely misreport date of birth, address, phone number, and events. Although technically, the onus is on the patient to make sure information provided to a facility corresponds with that in the records of the payer, the facility is left in most cases to act as a middle man if they want to maximize the amount of money they can collect for a particular interaction.

One aspect of contracting with payers that involves a lot of negotiating and administrative oversight is the so-called *capitation* contract. This is a contract with a payer that is based on a certain service volume, say 400 patient interactions per month, for which the facility receives a flat rate payment. If more patients than the capitated amount are seen in the contracted period, the facility is obligated to treat them on their own dime. If fewer are seen, the facility makes more revenue than they would have through individual, "fee for service" billing.

Payers and providers can use these types of contracts when they are engaged in a large volume of claims together and seek to normalize or hedge the common ebbs and flows while streamlining administrative overhead in the claims process. If used thoughtfully, this can be a boon to facilities and payers, but historically the more powerful analytics employed by payers have given them a distinct advantage.

Records

Historically, healthcare management has devoted a lot of effort to the physical aspects of medical record storage and retrieval. The collection of physical records, indexing, and coordination of records coming and going from other organizations has taken up a good deal of personnel mindshare. The gradual triumph of electronic records, driven forward partly by several explicit meaningful use requirements, upsets the historic balance of responsibility for records by eliminating the very need for such records at all and by systematizing the sharing of records in ways that providers can employ directly.

The impacts of the shift remain to be seen, but it should certainly result in cost savings. The overhead of employing staff solely to organize and physically move records, and the long-term costs of real estate devoted to storage of paper documents, will be eliminated and can be redirected to more productive avenues such as new space for patient care. Meaningful use is probably most lamented by photographers, who have long employed the overflowing medical records room as the iconic representation of the disorganized state of healthcare.

Demographics

Demographics are the minute details about patient records that distinguish them from other records and correlate people between the different parties we have covered in *the system*. Some demographics are very familiar, such as last name, first name, date of birth, and Social Security number, whereas other demographics are more obscure but still very important. Registration location, the first site in a multisite organization you presented to as a patient, details about race, ethnicity, and language, and other traits have become very important in understanding disparities in availability of care and the efficacy of certain treatments.

Healthcare management must collect, normalize, and organize all this data about patients. It is crucial first of all for clinical functions so that providers can be certain they are treating the correct patient. The billing department also depends on the demographic data because it appears on claims and must correspond very precisely with the patient details the payers have on file.

Meaningful use requires several demographics that are new to many facilities, including race, ethnicity, and preferred language. Those new details must be included in the reporting to meet meaningful use compliance.

Revenue Collection

Healthcare as a business does not differ all that much from other service industries when it comes to the difficulties of collecting balances owed on services delivered. We discussed complicating factors in Chapter 3. Some practices conduct their own collection operations, whereas others partner with a collection agency. Healthcare management is responsible for coordinating the activities with the general ledger and primary accounting operations.

Auditing

There is no shortage of agencies, partners, payers, and other authorities that seek to conduct audits of the practices and record-keeping of medical organizations. Healthcare management is ultimately responsible for preparing for audits and providing the necessary assistance during the audits. Statistical sampling of data is the most common kind of audit, to ensure that what has been previously reported has actually occurred in the numbers reported, and that records are free from tampering.

One of the more dreaded audits is that conducted by Medicare. They have perhaps the most opaque and voluminous rules and regulations and a reputation of being notably harsh when suspecting even unintentional fraud. For the most part, they have good reason to be tough. In June 2011, a $200 million scheme was unwound by Medicare fraud investigators in the Miami region, which involved unnecessary mental healthcare for patients who were coded, apparently unbeknownst to them, with fictitious diagnoses that qualified them for further treatment. That additional treatment was medically unnecessary but produced extensive additional billing. Already a 20-year jail sentence has been handed to a lead player who pled guilty, and several other arrests and settlements are pending. It would be inappropriate to call this an isolated incident. Fraud on this scale has unfortunately become a frequent occurrence for Medicare.

Accounting

Like any service business, healthcare firms have to conduct accounting for all of the overhead, salaries, hourly employees, and common business functions. Two primary differences come into play for healthcare. First the length of time that accounts receivable balances might be outstanding is typically longer than in almost any other industry. Second, medical billing has separate accounting from the general accounting that covers all other operations.

Reporting

A core business office role is producing operational, month-/quarter-end, and annual reporting for internal use and for communication to numerous payers, regulators, and programs. A lot of the reporting is created by legal or contractual requirements by outside parties. It generally includes line totals of specific patient interaction types, dollar totals, and breakouts by any or all of the demographic axes required as part of meaningful use. At a minimum, most facilities must file an annual state-level report, an annual federal-level report, and a report for each of the major payer contracts they have negotiated.

Facilities also create reports for various accounting measures that could be found in any business. A couple of reports specific to healthcare break out financial productivity by billing code (often called procedure productivity), payer productivity (to show disparities in compensation for specific billing codes by payer), percentage of no shows, and length of surgical procedures.

Meaningful use is a great opportunity for facilities to delve deeper into reporting and to combine healthcare management details with the clinical details newly found in the electronic clinical system. A very long running problem is that current billing data, in the form of billing codes, paints a very inaccurate picture when used in isolation for clinical review. Billing codes have little clinical value because of the hoops and machinations it takes to produce codes that will result in proper remuneration, and because of the codes' lack of specificity (there are only about 15,000 codes to cover the infinite number of treatments that could be delivered). Chapter 10 delves into that issue more comprehensively.

Meaningful use allows for an unprecedented marriage of practice management and clinical data, with much better accuracy and depth than in the past. A lot of basic questions in healthcare management that have remained largely unanswered can now be resolved in a straightforward manner. Examples where we are eager to start seeing high-quality data include which unexpected aspects of chronic diseases—such as obesity, diabetes, asthma, and high blood pressure—result in the most expensive aspects of treatment. Those chronic diseases encompass very large sets of symptoms and severity levels of disease that current billing coding captures very poorly. Detailed visit data, combined with information from healthcare management systems, will shed dramatic new light that can improve patient outcomes while also helping to better control costs.

Licensing, Credentials, and Enrollments

Even small facilities face a large undertaking to ensure that providers have the proper paperwork and records to practice medicine within the municipal, state, and federal environment. Medical facilities are situated in very complicated legal environments involving municipal regulations on zoning, disposal of waste, occupancy, and electrical use. It is the responsibility of the administrative staff to keep up with all the regulatory filing and responses. From a personnel standpoint, healthcare involves many more layers than other industries. Specifically, providers have numerous licensing and on-going education requirements. The process of keeping track of those requirements and coordinating the ongoing education is generally referred to as *credentialing*. Providers of all types must be licensed in the states where they are practicing by a state medical board, after passing a state testing procedure.

Once licensed, providers must complete additional education each year and earn what is called *continuing medical education* (CME) credits. In theory, CME is intended to keep providers up to date on the latest advancements within relevant research and standards in their specialties. In practice, a lot of CME programs and events take place in Hawaii or near U.S. Open golf courses. We'll leave it to the reader to determine the relative benefits of this process. In any case, healthcare management involves keeping on top of CME and licensing requirements to make sure that providers have met all necessary legal requirements to treat.

With much the same diligence, attention must be paid to equipment and spaces within a facility to ensure legal use: physical plant inspections of operating theaters, specialty inspection and repair of gas supply systems, physicist calibrations of imaging equipment, and a plethora of other medically unique repair, maintenance, and service tasks.

For each payer that a facility might bill, the business office must complete paperwork to enroll providers or the facility as a participating organization before it can actually bill the payer. The paperwork involved is never simple and can be quite voluminous if many providers and payers are involved, with at least one individual enrollment contract occurring between each combination of payer and provider.

Larger facilities often engage in very complex negotiations with payers over the compensation for specific billing codes. Occasionally this boils over and receives national attention in a high-stakes game of chicken. A particularly drawn-out dispute happened in Florida in 2010 between a regional hospital associated with 18 facilities covering most of the patient service area in major cities and United Healthcare, which insured roughly 400,000 patients in that region.

Nonhealthcare Interactions

A lot of interactions can happen in a healthcare facility that have little or even nothing to do with health or healthcare at all. When patients lack sufficient funds or coverage from third-party payers, the business office must complete a lot of research and paperwork to generate alternative funding. Different facilities handle this in different ways through an administrative staffer, a social worker, or sometimes the providers themselves.

Many healthcare facilities also serve nonhealthcare service roles in many communities, delivering social work, employment assistance, and youth programs in addition to healthcare. Many types of healthcare organizations themselves are hybrids of non-healthcare companies that serve general social purposes, including religious service, disease-specific advocacy agencies, and all of the myriad types of programs we reviewed in Chapter 3.

The Evolution of the Business Office

Healthcare administration, as we have seen, suffers from an odd nexus of traditional business responsibilities, unique requirements as a result of healthcare's peculiarities, and a sometimes antagonistic relationship with clinical departments based on mutual need. Meaningful use is a game changer that introduces many new opportunities for efficiency, cost control, and the improvement of patient outcomes, but also upsets the traditional apple cart in an industry not known for rapid change. The dollar signs attached to meaningful use glean a lot of the spotlight when it comes to talk among administrators, but it must be said that anyone seeking to profit from meaningful use incentives is sorely misled. The hard costs and organizational disruptions embodied in meaningful use compliance are profound, and the incentive payments are by no means certain, but the label for those payments could not be clearer: *incentive*. The incentives offered are a prodding by the federal government to private organizations to take this as an opportunity and get ahead of pending requirements and penalties. Facilities that miss this opportunity will be at a severe disadvantage in the in the years to come.

CHAPTER 6

Patient-Facing Software

Applications and web tools to engage patients and healthy people are potentially the most exciting facet of health IT. This type of software, when designed and used well, can be a source of tremendous patient empowerment. And the patient experience needs a radical transformation, because—in case you have never dealt with an extensive illness—being a patient can be demoralizing, frustrating, and humiliating. The unsettling burden of serious illness is often augmented by the task of coordinating care between various institutions, a task forced on many patients and caregivers.

The more complex a patient's condition, and the more experts that a patient has consulted, the more difficult the coordination of care becomes. Any person who frequents hospitals has seen the poor souls for whom this has become a Herculean task. They are easy to spot. They usually carry a travel briefcase, complete with rollers. The briefcase contains copies of all the patient records they have accumulated as they meander through the healthcare system. The healthcare system in the United States is easily one of the best in the world, until you need more than one doctor. A single doctor in the United States has met one of the highest standards for medical education in the world, but the system as a whole has been operating in a disconnected fashion for decades. Patients have been forced to coordinate their own care, and when a medical record is paper-based, this can be a daunting task indeed.

Two technologies together should make the process of coordinating care much simpler. One of them is the Nation Wide Health Information Network, which will become the Health Internet (discussed later in Chapter 11), and the other is patient-facing health records. Both of these approaches are required by meaningful use. Moreover, many meaningful use requirements will become much easier to accomplish using personal health records (PHRs) or PHR-like extensions to hospital and clinic technology.

Remember when we were trying to decide how to parse the names for EHRs? PHR terminology has dilemmas of its own. It is difficult to know just what should qualify as a PHR.

The names for patient-facing software solutions are varied and controversial. Most people refer to patient-facing healthcare software as PHRs. Some people insist that they should be called PCHRs, or personally controlled health records. This distinction was particularly important in the early days of PHR development. Many PHR systems were simply viewers for patients into their own record inside an EHR system maintained by the institution they were visiting. The patients could see and copy the data, but they could not modify, create, or even comment on the data inside the system. The term PCHR was emphasized as a way to distinguish this "window PHR model" from systems that were under the control and direction of the patient.

It is not clear how, or even if, PHR software is different from EHR software. The Tolven project is an open source health record that has two interfaces, one for patients and one for healthcare providers (doctors, nurses, etc.). The Tolven project holds that the healthcare record should be stored in one software system, and that the difference between a PHR and EHR is merely a question of what users have what privileges.

But most people assume that PHR software should be separate from EHR software, and as a result, it usually is.

There are two popular PHR configurations. In the "tethered" model, a body that controls a repository of patient data opens up that data to the patients in question. Patients' queries or changes to the PHR get passed through to the data source and display the data found there, allowing patients to modify and generate data to different degrees. The tethered PHR has often been guilty of the window PHR design. Even when tethered PHRs allowed patients to enter and change data, they created yet another silo of disconnected patient data.

Usually tethered PHR systems are offered by hospitals or clinics, but insurance companies, pharmacies, lab test companies, and countless other organizations have patient data and release that information directly to the patient through PHR systems. Most common tethered PHRs are web applications. As an experiment, you might take a moment to discover just how many PHR systems already provide you with access to your own healthcare data. You can expect one from each insurance company, one from each large hospital you have visited, and still another if you are a veteran covered by the VA.

The other historical model for PHR systems has been the stand-alone PHR. This allows consumers to enter their own clinical data, and organize and manage that data online. During the dot-com boom, many stand-alone PHR vendors received funding from venture capitalists. Most of the dot-com PHR companies went out of business once the venture capital ran out. Business plans based on assumptions that patients would pay for the privilege of performing data entry of their own health data failed. Most commercial PHR systems now assume that patients should not need to pay for the PHR service, and that data entry be kept to a minimum. When manual data is required from the users, modern PHR services ensure that something of substantial value to the patient is delivered as a result of that data entry. Mere classification and structure is not enough to motivate most patients to enter health data manually into a PHR system.

Although the difference between tethered and untethered or stand-alone has become entrenched in modern parlance, both are based on assumptions that are no longer true. Most important, it is no longer a reasonable assumption that movement of data from EHR to PHR should be one-way. Both the siloed PHR with no integration with anything and the tethered PHR with only the capacity to import data from an EHR are largely dead concepts. Modern thinking about PHRs presumes that useful data should flow bidirectionally between PHR and EHR systems. In the last decade it was a good assumption that data in an EHR either was generated by local clinical users of that EHR or imported from some other EHR, but over the next decade this will become a bad assumption. EHR users and technicians should carefully consider this chapter, because soon the data sent to PHRs will automatically appear in your EHR systems. Even if you are not directly working with a PHR, you will probably need to deal with PHR-sourced data.

Meaningful use will be interpreted as a mandate for tethered PHR systems at a minimum, but both the tethered and stand-alone models will soon be left behind by more advanced PHR deployment models that defy easy categorization. The first such model is the PHR platform.

The PHR as Platform

The two dominant PHR platforms are Microsoft HealthVault and Indivo X. Google Health had been a dominant platform, but as of June 2011, Google retired the Google Health project and will no longer offer a PHR.

When Google and Microsoft decided to enter the PHR market, it spelled the end of the already struggling dot-com startups that had focused on developing stand-alone PHR systems. Microsoft HealthVault was released in 2007 and Google announced Google Health in 2008. Both Microsoft and Google announced that they would not only be developing a costless consumer-facing PHR product, but would also be releasing an integration layer for the PHR systems. They invited third-party developers to offer new and interesting functionality on top of their basic functionality and invited healthcare data sources such as hospitals and clinics to upload data on particular patients using the same interfaces.

Philosophically the technical approaches could not have been more different, or more indicative of the different technical styles of the two companies.

Microsoft designed HealthVault to support almost any reasonable health data operation, including the storage of digital data and arbitrary data types. You can upload medical images studies to HealthVault, for instance. Most important, HealthVault includes extensive libraries for embedded applications. Microsoft knows how to develop the software that runs devices and created a Software Development Kit that allows its software to be easily embedded directly into computers and devices that gather healthcare data, as long as those devices are running either a Microsoft operating system or are near a Microsoft computer. HealthVault extends the Microsoft Windows Portable Device architecture to support health and wellness data. The notion is that if a device manufacturer interfaces at a low level with the Microsoft operating system, they can leverage that interface for simple HealthVault PHR connectivity.

HealthVault has had an interesting relationship with the Open Source health IT community. Microsoft promised to release the specification for the HealthVault application programming interface (API) under Open Source friendly licenses. Originally, they had intended to release the HealthVault API specification under the Microsoft Open Specification Promise (OSP). This is a strong promise that was created, as part of the European antitrust compromises, for the open source Samba project to have access to protocol specifications. Ultimately, Microsoft did release the specification, but under a much less generous specification license. So far, no Open Source implementation of the HealthVault API exists. Microsoft has been criticized for its protocol licensing, but Google Health, its main competitor, has no mention of protocol licensing at all. This issue has been critical now that Google is abandoning all of the companies who invested in their API. Given how badly these organizations have fared with the retirement of Google Health, both of these interface standards are likely to be mildly interesting historical footnotes, as we move toward well-adopted open standards for healthcare interoperability. The Direct Project (see "The Direct Project/Protocol" on page 198), now that it has support as Google's mechanism for allowing users to migrate, will likely become the default PHR integration API.

The notion of presenting a proprietary API for PHR platform integration made perfect sense in the age before meaningful use. Now it is apparent that standard and open protocols will be at the heart of future health IT integration. This progression would never have been possible without the interchange requirements of meaningful use, and the strong position that Office of the National Coordinator (ONC), the shepherd of the meaningful use standard, has taken with respect to health data exchange protocols. Because of this, standards like the Integrating the Healthcare Enterprise (IHE) and Direct, which are discussed fully in Chapter 11, will likely serve to connect EHR systems with PHR systems like Google Health or Microsoft HealthVault.

Surprisingly, one of the most significant contributions that Microsoft, or anyone for that matter, has made to health IT has been toward an open source project. The Direct Project is a critical piece of what will become the Health Internet. Contrary to Microsoft's typical stance on open source, the HealthVault team was active in the project from the beginning, strongly advocated for open source values (i.e., simplicity and equality) during critical decision points on the Direct Project, and created an open source .NET implementation of Direct that, alongside the Java implementation, enabled the first proof of concept of the Direct networks. Microsoft has bet far more heavily on the Direct Project than Google Health, and is the first PHR system to offer Direct addresses to the public at large.

The Direct protocol, and its companion protocol IHE, together make the question of integration somewhat moot, but rich APIs are still going to be important in the PHR platform space. The Direct protocol is focused on super-simple point-to-point health data interchange, whereas IHE is primarily focused on the complexities of health data exchange between healthcare institutions. There remains an unmet need for a set of interfaces for applications to provide cutting-edge functionality between third-party patient systems and PHR platforms. Given the unclear nature of API licensing available from both Google and Microsoft, a third platform, Indivo X, will probably prove to be the dominant API platform for interfacing between patient facing health information systems.

Google Health released an API that centered on a subset of the Continuity of Care Record (CCR), which is a clean, relatively simple XML-based standard for healthcare records that we discuss further in Chapter 11. Google embedded the CCR content inside an ATOM feed. ATOM is an XML standard for changing the content of a target document that receives the feed. ATOM is an upgrade to the more familiar RSS, an XML standard that allows for the easy parsing of the contents of blogs. ATOM is used more generally for tracking any kind of constantly updating data. It is unclear at this stage what will become of the Google Health API. Although this might change soon, at the time of the writing there are no plans to release Google Health as open source or to release the Google Health API as an open API standard.

Google Health will probably have more influence on the PHR market in the way that it ended than with anything else it has ever done. In the blog post that announced the retirement of Google Health, Google endorsed both Microsoft HealthVault and, more important, the Direct Project as a transfer to migrate data out of Google Health:

> Over the coming weeks we'll also be adding the ability to directly transfer your health data to other services that support the Direct Project protocol, an emerging open standard for efficient health data exchange. And while we'll discontinue the Google Health service at the beginning of 2012, we'll keep these download options available for one more year, through the start of 2013. This approach to download and transfer capability is part of Google's strong commitment to data liberation principles: providing free and easy ways for users to maintain control of their data and move it out of Google's services at any time.

Ironically, this was the first formal announcement from Google Health that they would be supporting the Direct Project protocol. By the time that Google Health supports Direct-based export, there will probably be several PHR systems that support Direct-based import. However, Microsoft HealthVault was the first provider to launch publicly available Direct addresses (Direct is essentially a secure email protocol focused on delivering clinical data) and was the only PHR service specifically mentioned in the Google Health retirement announcement as a viable alternative.

Indivo X is the latest iteration of one of the longest standing PHR development efforts in the world. Work on predecessors of Indivo date back to 1994. Both Google Health and HealthVault had the benefit of developing while the lessons and source code from early versions of Indivo were available. The industry regards the Indivo project as the grandfather of PHR systems.

In 2006 a group of employers decided that their employees might benefit from access to a PHR system. They concluded, correctly, that most people would not be comfortable with the notion that their employers had easy access to their complete health record. As a result, several large employers, including such giants as AT&T, BP, Intel, and Walmart, created a foundation called Dossia. Dossia decided to use the Java version of the Indivo system as the basis for their PHR platform. This was a tremendous vote of confidence for the Indivo team, which was already deep into the third generation of its PHR development.

The latest iteration of Indivo is called Indivo X, and is obviously a fourth-generation effort in the PHR arena. The genesis of the design made a tremendous splash with an perspective article in the *New England Journal of Medicine* in 2009.[1]

The Indivo team advocated for deeper investment in several principles for PHR platforms, specifically evoking the effective model that the iPhone app store was just pioneering. The article laid out several principles that are deeply ingrained in the architecture of Indivo X:

Liquidity of data
    The platform should not introduce impediments to the open flow of data.

Substitutability of applications
    The platform should support subapplications that should be replaceable by the end user. So if you do not like your blood pressure module, you should be able to replace it with a better (for you) module.

Built on open standards
    Friendly to both open source and proprietary software and licenses.

Support for a peer-to-peer PHR instance model
    Multiple instances of Indivo X are expected to be installed and effectively operate separately, cooperating to make data liquid between Indivo X instances. This principle is not specifically mentioned in the article, but can be deduced as a major goal of the project.

Indivo X offers a platform for applications. In itself, Indivo X provides a data storage facility and an API. The applications are responsible for providing everything seen by the patient or clinician who is entering or consuming the health data, whether it be a mobile app, a web interface, or data exchange with a medical device. Indivo X is built using Python, but provides the current standard for programming interfaces—a RESTful API—to allow applications to be written in almost any language.

Although both the Google Health and Microsoft HealthVault platforms support some of these principles, or to some extent even all of the principles here, only the Indivo X platform has been architected to embody these notions fully.

---

1. No Small Change for the Health Information Economy (*http://www.nejm.org/doi/full/10.1056/NEJMp0900411*)

Recently, the Indivo team has been trying to take many of the same concepts embodied inside Indivo X and extend them to a more general health IT application. That effort is called the SMART platform (*http://www.smartplatforms.org*) and has received both funding and attention from the U.S. government and other major healthcare players. Eventually the principles behind Indivo X and SMART could lead to a radically different notion of how health IT should be architected generally. Currently, SMART is very new, but Indivo X has established itself as one of the three dominant PHR platforms, and the leading open source PHR project.

Sharing Data in Patient-Facing Software

One of the most difficult challenges for any patient-facing system is whether and how to allow sharing between its users. Most people simply do not care that much about their privacy, as evidenced by their utter lack of outrage toward Facebook, which regularly flouts its ability to change its privacy policies and privacy architecture. But most people view Facebook as part of the public sphere, and make different assumptions regarding their health information. For the most part, PHR systems place greater technical controls on the exchange of health information. Users must make obvious and significant choices when they decide to share with other users.

We will discuss issues related to children having PHR records, and the laws that cover PHR systems in the discussion of health IT regulations LINK. But for now it is enough to know that most typical PHR systems, especially the platforms already mentioned, have spent considerable energy ensuring basic privacy functionality.

Patients Using Normal Social Media

A new category of software for patients appeals specifically to people who would rather share generously than have specific privacy controls. Many of these sites support different forms of open discussion between patients. Often, users participate in these discussions using their real names, but using pseudonyms is also popular. A pseudonym usually takes the form of a username that cannot be mapped to any real name. If people participate in an online patient community with the names ftrotter and duhlman, they can easily be mapped to real-world identities. But usernames like ThatGuyInHouston or ItsADryHeat help protect the "real-life" identity of patient community participants.

People who embraced public or semipublic discussion of their own health care started with the same technologies that built the initial phases of communication and collaboration on the Internet, forums and mailing lists.

The grandfather of all patient hubs is ACOR, the Association of Cancer Online Resources (*http://www.acor.org*). This mailing list has tremendously knowledgeable patients, patient advocates, patient caregivers, and even doctors who often provide more specialized information regarding available cancer therapies than most doctors are aware of. At least that was the experience of Dave deBronkart.

E-patient Dave,[2] as he is now affectionately known, was diagnosed with metastasized stage IV cancer (*http://epatientdave.com/book/*) (that's "bad" for my geek readers). By following advice from the ACOR mailing lists, Dave was able to find a treatment that cured him. Dave's experience was especially interesting because if he had followed the standard treatment path, his chances would have been substantially poorer and he would have disqualified himself for the experimental treatment that ultimately worked for him. Dave brings an engineering approach to being a patient that should appeal to any geek. His book is both readable and relevant for anyone who wants to engage seriously in health IT.

But e-patient Dave did not gain notoriety for his ability to effectively navigate the healthcare system. In fact it was his online review of his experience using Google Health that ultimately lead to his fame in health IT. Some people have taken to calling his experience "e-patient Dave-gate." He wrote a detailed blog post (*http://patientdave .blogspot.com/2009/04/imagine-someone-had-been-managing-your.html*) that showed the strange errors caused by the import of his medical record from Beth Israel Deaconess Medical Center (BIDMC) into Google Health. These errors were focused on how Google and BIDMC relied on medical billing data as reliable clinical information. Several of the Google Health integrations, including pharmacy integrations, have had this issue (*http://groups.google.com/group/googlehealthdevelopers/browse_thread/thread/ d4e0f6cd8643284f/6383805ea69c8da6?lnk=gst&q=cvs&pli=1*).

Back to ACOR. ACOR is based on very old Internet technologies. It is basically a garden-variety combination of mailing lists with online archives. What was revolutionary about ACOR was how it was being used, not the technology that powered it.

Each subsequent improvement in the Internet's capacity to allow people to connect with each other and to allow patient-to-patient support has been fully embraced by a vibrant subset of patients who, as we've seen, refer to themselves as "e-patients." Modern social media outlets, especially, have generated a movement to allow patients to empower themselves by communicating and educating each other using. Patient communities have become common on Facebook. Often, more specialized social media tools, like Ning (which allows you to set up a miniature social network) have been specifically leveraged to set up targeted patient communities. A useful experiment is to search Twitter for specialized patient content like #paralysis (*http://twitter.com/ #search?q=%23paralysis*) or #multiplesclerosis (*http://twitter.com/#search?q= %23multiplesclerosis*).

Watch your friends' posts to Facebook carefully. Often your connections will be using Facebook to log their health experience. Here are modified and deidentified Facebook posts from a person who is attending the Mayo Clinic for nerve damage:

---

2. The e stands for "empowered" as well as "electronic."

I'm super sick today. Also please pray for my blood pressure & heart rate to become normal - they're running low this morning. I'll be glad when I am able to post something other than health stuff in my status.

Mayo diagnosed me when I was 16. The nerve damage to my organs is why I have so many health issues. My trips to the Mayo clinic are for monitoring organs and addressing new issues with them. My husband & I have beautiful goals for our life. In "sickness & health" ... We are blessed. Xoxo

So tired of the pain and nausea... :(I can either just suffer or turn my sufferings into something amazing that wouldn't be otherwise. So I'm off to write...

Had a rough week. Stomach is bleeding. More diagnostic tests tomorrow. Praying now, because I'm physically done.

Of course, her friends responded with encouragement and offers for support. What is important here is the mix of health data with social and spiritual content. This person is using Facebook as a kind of practical catharsis; chronicling her condition, coordinating her care with her support network, and having a kind of public prayer journal. Facebook is the medium, but this is clearly health data, sometimes extremely specific. These journal entries have been anonymized and changed substantially in this book, but this person has recorded this information with little regard for her privacy. Given the size of her social network, and the way Facebook extends posts to friends of friends, she is effectively publishing her health details to a population equivalent to a small rural town.

E-patients

The e-patient movement has that moniker precisely because the community recognizes that their use of "electronic" tools has an empowering effect. The e-patient movement, which is loosely organized around a blog (*http://e-patient.net*), a whitepaper (*http://e-patients.net/e-Patients_White_Paper.pdf*), and a nonprofit, the Society for Participatory Medicine (*http://participatorymedicine.org/*), is focused on technologies that improve the ability of patients to engage in their own care.

There are a surprising number of resources available to patients on the Internet now regarding health information. Of course it is obligatory to mention sites like WebMD that have become standards of information that patients can leverage to gain information about health-related issues. But very often there are resources that go beyond the overview that these type of sites offer. Sometimes these resources are dangerous, as evidenced by the compelling "tale of two e-patients" (*http://www.youtube.com/watch?v=9ebdGR3IZp8*), but this danger is commonly vastly overestimated. Good research shows that typical search results on health topics on the popular Internet search engines typically return solid health information (which is constantly improving). Patient communities have very low error rates, and generally self-correct when they do have bad information.[3]

E-patients typically have tastes for deeper levels of information than are available on "for public consumption" health information websites. Invariably, websites like WebMD offer an accurate summary of a health issue, but then end with something like "Be sure to ask your doctor....". That phrase is generally evidence that the resource in question is intentionally abdicating any attempt to be an in-depth resource on a given health subject. In many cases, a patient is seeking to correct the fundamental information asymmetry in health care. Is the surgeon recommending surgery for me because it is what is best for my care, or because he gets paid $2,000 every time he conducts surgery? If an e-patient is trying to evaluate a doctor or doctors, ending with "Ask your doctor" is particularly unhelpful. What e-patients want is access to the same information that the doctor has. More and more, that information is available. In many cases, there are services that help nonclinicians parse the information on a particular procedure or condition that is aimed at doctors.

Wikipedia is surprisingly useful for this. Wikipedia has become more and more stringent in the standards for articles, and health or medicine-related articles receive constant attention. A large part of recent improvements to Wikipedia's articles include more numerous and accurate references. A Wikipedia search on any subject will link to articles in the *New England Journal of Medicine* (NEJM), the *Journal of the American Medical Association* (JAMA), or Pubmed, precisely the type of resources that are aimed at doctors, and just the sort of thing e-patients crave.[4]

But Wikipedia is just the beginning of new and innovate ways for patients to become hyperinformed about medical issues. Up To Date (*http://www.uptodate.com*) is an expensive service that provides doctors with the most recent scientific consensus around a particular health issue. It now has an offering specifically designed to enable patients temporary and inexpensive access to the same information (*http://www.xmlmind.com/ xmleditor/namespace/clipboard" ><!--http://www.cautiouspatient.org/blog/item/47-re alities-of-medical-care-series-45-of-patients-get-only-partially-treated.html*). This resource is perfect for patients who only want to know lots of information about one or two issues in any case.

The Quantified Self

Other patients are seeking to gain new information advantages in a different way. Participants in the quantified self (or quantters) movement seek to improve their health by obsessively measuring anything they can. In centuries past, there were a few cases of individuals given over to a deep desire to record and journal every aspect of their

---

3. Accuracy and Self Correction of Information Received from an Internet Breast Cancer List: Content Analysis (*http://www.ncbi.nlm.nih.gov/pubmed/16513686*)

4. Wikipedia's health information has also been found to be high quality (*http://www.bivings.com/thelab/ presentations/Wikipedia_Health_Information.pdf*).

---

lives. Today, a much less obsessed individual can automatically record far more data about himself using digital devices.

Quantters use smartphones to track many different kinds of things, but are also willing to purchase specialized devices that record specific information. Fitbit (*http://www.fit bit.com*) is an accelerometer that can track almost any type of movement (an advancement over the pedometer, which only records steps). The Zeo (*http://www.myzeo .com*) is a device that tracks your sleep patterns. Over-the-counter glucose monitors can provide simple access to glucose data and, using USB interfaces, upload it to a computer. With a prescription it is possible to get a glucose monitor that you wear all the time, providing the kind of near-real-time data feed that quantters crave. Another device, the Withings scale, allows users to automatically broadcast their weight to Twitter and Facebook each time they step on the scale. The list of manufacturers that provide consumer-oriented healthcare data devices offering direct integration with multiple online data sources will continue to grow. In a few years each of these devices, which are now very unique, will be product categories with several competitors.

Many quantters pipe the data feeds from these devices to Twitter, which has become a data layer of choice for real time-health data. When there is no device to record data, quantters can use parser-friendly syntaxes like ohme (*http://code.google.com/p/omhe*) to write data about what they ate or an analog measurement they just took, knowing that a parser can later quantify the time-stamped data. Ohme is an example of a *micro-syntax*, which allows very dense healthcare information to be stored in a very small space.

Soon inexpensive accelerometer technologies will enable the movement associated with any object to be tracked and quantified. It will become possible to place a sticker on your toothbrush containing an embedded accelerometer that tracks the movement of the toothbrush and automatically uploads the data to the Internet. It is not too far-fetched to imagine that soon your toothbrush will be communicating directly with your PHR record, which might automatically forward that information directly to your dentist.

For instance, the Withings scale integrates directly with HealthVault. Although the most extreme quantified self practices will probably never take hold in the general population, real-time health and fitness data will soon become a natural part of EHR and PHR systems. Some of the most avid quantters are e-patients who seek to use hyperaccurate information about their asthma attacks, migraine headaches, or just random pain to discover and eliminate the unexpected causes. The Robert Wood Johnson Foundation, one of the most important funding foundations for healthcare informatics, has specifically funded projects oriented toward recording observations of daily living (ODLs). For those who suffer chronic pain of any kind, information about what "sets off" the pain is crucial for a normal lifestyle.

The types of devices and data sources continue to expand, blending entertainment, social media, and healthcare IT. EA Sports, a video game company, has released a heart monitor that integrates with video game consoles like the Microsoft Xbox and the Nintendo Wii. This, in combination with the ability of the game consoles to accurately capture movements using devices like the Microsoft Kinect, will provide hyperaccurate fitness data that has never been available before. Is the EA Sports application a video game that requires movement, or a special-purpose PHR system? The answer is probably "yes."

Perhaps the most relevant information that such devices will soon generate is compliance data. Generally, the word compliance is shortened from compliant with doctors instructions. It should be obvious how systems already in use by the quantified self community could be used to measure compliance with diet and exercise instructions. But even more concerning to clinicians is medicine compliance. Patients suffer when they fail to take medications properly, but often they are not the only ones hurt. The ongoing battle to prevent the spread of resistant bacteria is hampered by patients who stop taking antibiotics after they "feel better." Failure to comply with medicinal treatment plan is an expensive problem. Currently, the best source of compliance data is medicine refill data. If a person refills a prescription regularly, it is a reasonable assumption that he or she is taking the medication properly.

In the future, there will be no reason to make this assumption. There are two approaches that are already in limited use that will track medication adherence far more accurately. The first is a device that replaces a medicine bottle cap with a sensor that can tell when the medicine bottle is being opened. Of course this device cannot tell how much was taken at a given time, but it can tell the schedule when the medicine bottle was opened. In the future, tiny radio devices will be embedded inside pills that will allow each pill to be accurately tracked through a patient's digestive system. These types of personal data quantification will allow healthcare providers to have hyperaccurate measurements of patient compliance.

Social media, advanced gaming, and the capacity for devices to automatically gather a huge depth of data truly is a paradigm shift in health IT.

Patient-Focused Social Media

Perhaps the most interesting use of social media in healthcare are the new generations of applications that blend the definitions of PHR and social network. This new generation of consumer-facing applications, often under the flag of Health 2.0, is giving patients condition-specific tools to track their healthcare data and then share it in a social context.

Patients Like Me (*http://www.patientslikeme.com*) is emblematic of this new type of application. Patients Like Me provides health data tools in a social media context that are targeted toward patients with a particular condition. For instance, in the HIV positive patient community at Patients Like Me, you can review a person's history of CD4 cell/mm, CD4 percent, and viral load. Patients with severe life-altering conditions usually have more than one, especially depression, which almost all patients with serious conditions must battle at one time or another. Patients Like Me allows patients to connect with other patients who are going through the same things they are. If an ALS patient is considering intensive outpatient group therapy for treatment of depression, he or she can find out what another ALS patient thought of that option after having taken the therapy.

Patients Like Me is a leader in the field, but it is hardly without competition. There are several other websites that are offering similar services.

You will find that health IT "experts" like to make definitive statements about PHR systems (and health IT systems generally), but when you consider a system like Patients Like Me, Xbox Kinect, or even Facebook as a PHR system, it becomes obvious that patient-facing health IT is moving faster than our convenient categorizations for them can keep up. As with other subjects in health IT, the most important thing to learn from this section is that there is more than one way to reasonably approach the same set of problems.

Patient Privacy in PHR Systems

For some people, a full discussion of the types of data that will and are being gathered on individuals is always uncomfortable. It is really not possible to discuss these technological improvements without considering privacy, but we consider it last because it is difficult to consider privacy without understanding just how much data is going to be generated.

Practitioners tend to disagree on what patient privacy means, or what the implications are. As we have seen in this chapter, a new generation of patients think nothing of publishing everything about themselves online for the whole world to watch. They have learned something that many in older generations do not yet understand. For the most part, publishing health information online is perfectly safe because no one is paying attention. Or rather, the attention that publicly posted health data gets is general use for data mining purposes. It is used to make conclusions about populations rather than conclusions about individuals.

For the most part, the public is excellent at ignoring health data of any kind. If you are unlucky enough to have a serious medical condition, and you decided to publish this information on the Internet, you would have a very difficult time getting people to even notice that the information was there. Many people choose to blog or tweet about their healthcare and only the very best and frequent writers are able to maintain even a small audience. Publishing your health information on the Internet does not typically matter because the Internet audience does not care about you or your health information. Your health insurance company has so much data about you that it cannot fully process it. Currently, insurance companies are probably not going to go to your Facebook page and look at your posts.

This will change, and perhaps soon. Insurance companies make more money when they correctly identify an individual as a high risk. In any insurance market, if insurance companies can develop a substantial evaluation advantage over their competitors, they have the temptation to "cherry pick," providing insurance only to those who are very unlikely to ever need it. Hopefully, insurance regulations will make such cherry picking impossible before patients' social media postings and full purchasing history are used to exclude them from insurance coverage.

The best way to solve the problem of health insurance company privacy violations is to negate the financial benefit of gathering the information. This was one of the goals of the health insurance reforms put in place under President Obama. Hopefully these changes will help ensure that health insurance companies do not have a financial incentive to use social media or PHR data against insurers. If it is not prevented at a policy level, it is reasonable to assume that data that you post about yourself on Facebook or Twitter, or even what you buy using your credit cards, could someday be used to determine your health insurance rates.

The real difficult issues of privacy have nothing to do with the Internet and everything to do with your personal relationships. Many people want to keep specific details about their health from their spouse, their parents, or their employers. PHR systems are designed to share information only with those whom you authorize. Most PHR architectures, including all three of the major platforms that are mentioned here, spend a tremendous amount of time making sure that the information does not "leak" onto the public Internet.

But personal privacy, especially among family members, is very difficult with PHR systems. It is a little easier to exclude employers, who are already excluded from most health care data by default.

Let's imagine a spouse who has contracted a minor sexually transmitted disease (STD). The law (HIPAA) says that the patient can expect that fact to be entirely private information between the patient and the medical staff. Previously the couple had used a tethered PHR system offered by the hospital to get lab results back. Both wife and husband had access to each other's accounts using the sharing function. When one member of the couple discovers an STD as the result on an infidelity, that person would want to be able to either exclude that data from his or her PHR, or find a way to disable the access that the spouse previously had to his or her PHR record. Either or both should be enabled by smart filters at the interface between the PHR and the EHR, and by careful filtering between data elements on a PHR chart. This is a fragile situation. It is easy for an "unrelated" data point to slip through and compromise the secret. For instance, imagine the "in-the-dark" spouse reading on the PHR record about a mysterious "appointment" at the clinic, or perhaps an automated appointment reminder phone call that the "in-the-dark" spouse intercepts. The simplest way to avoid these types of problems is to detect when this type of problem might occur, and move to human-to-human voice-only communication regarding the issue. But even this can be problematic. Imagine a dialogue beginning, "Honey, why does Jane call us for every appointment reminder now, and why can't I log in to the PHR anymore..." Tricky stuff indeed.

PHR/EHR systems with adequate privacy and security controls can mitigate these risks, but most health staff are not trained well enough on the software to understand how to filter data carefully. Over the next few years, as health data generally becomes more liquid, we're likely to see more and more slip-ups that are attributable not to the technology itself, but rather to lack of familiarity with the technology.

The other patient data access issue that is worth mentioning explicitly is children. A favorite quote from a friend who is the CIO of my local children's hospital is, "In health IT, children are not just short adults."

Divorces, child abuse, teen pregnancy, and countless other child and teen-related health IT issues will be very difficult to get right over the coming years. Most PHR systems assume that sometime during the teen years (the particular trigger varies across states), patients gain the right to have health data privacy from their parents. Often this change can be the result of an event (teen pregnancy or HIV status change) rather than an age. This is a very difficult area to automate, because state laws vary dramatically on what rights children and parents have at given times.

Soon, access to child's PHR might be an item negotiated in divorce settlements. For now, when both parents of a divorced child have access to a shared PHR record for a child, information about treatment for a broken arm can become evidence in competence hearings. Of course, if a child was being abused by a step-parent, then the parent without custody perhaps should have a right to information such as ER visits. Who gets to see the information, and what they get to do with it, are difficult decisions made on a case-by-case basis. These are just a few of the issues that will make children's or pediatric hospitals and clinics typically late PHR adopters.

Privacy advocates sometimes give in to fear mongering over their chosen issue, but most Americans are far more concerned about too little data liquidity than too much.[5]

In fact, in the future, PHRs will become a critical means for patients to manage this data liquidity. Many if not most health records have errors. Sometimes these errors are simply the presence of discarded diagnoses that were temporarily used for billing purposes. Sometimes the errors are far more serious, such as missing or extra allergies or incorrect medications or dosing. When health data becomes more liquid, data integrity will become a far greater problem than patient privacy. In the future PHR or PCHR systems will be the central way for patients to combat health misinformation in an automated fashion.

---

5. "Privacy concerns may take back seat" (*http://www.modernhealthcare.com/article/20110321/NEWS/303219928?AllowView=VW8xUmo5Q21TcWJOb1gzb0tNN3RLZ0h0MWg5SVgra3NZRzROR3l0WWRMZmJWLzhBRWxiNUtpQzMyWmVvNVgwWUpiNnA=*) by David Burda, March 21, 2011.

Specific PHR and Patient-Directed Meaningful Use Requirements

There are several stages of meaningful use requirements related to PHRs. Rather than discuss the current revision here, which will soon be out of date, we list the fundamental areas that relate to patient-facing health IT systems.

Patient reminders and preventative care notices could include text messages, automated phone calls, emails, messages through the Direct network, or contact through the PHR. There are HIPAA concerns regarding health data sent across insecure channels, but text messages and emails that simply say "Call us" or "Log in to the PHR" should be fine. There is also a specific requirement to support secure patient messaging (i.e., Direct) and to record and respect the patient's preferred means of digital communication.

Regarding direct patient access to data inside an EHR system, there are several meaningful use requirements for access through a system that sounds very much like a tethered PHR. The software must be able to provide a complete copy of electronic health information on request, specifically the ability to view recent data through a web portal soon after discharge. Patients will need to be able to browse and filter data, even if that data did not originate from within the clinic or hospital that is offering the web portal. Patients will need to be able to download this in human readable (e.g., a PDF) and digital (e.g., CCD/CCR) formats.

To achieve comprehensive certification, EHR vendors must be able to support all of the core and menu-set meaningful use requirements. Given that, most EHR systems will have simple tethered PHR options. These PHR components vary wildly in quality and style. A clinic or hospital could also simply support EHR-to-Direct patient record requests and allow stand-alone PHR systems like HealthVault to handle the user interface. Of course, for an arrangement like this to work, HealthVault will need to become certified as a provider of these patient-facing features. Eventually, communication with nontethered PHR systems over a health information network of some kind will likely be required as well. Others, such as psychiatric hospitals, which are especially concerned with privacy, will simply provide copies of electronic files to a patient face-to-face.

Some aspects of meaningful use are focused on providing patient education using automated systems. For instance, patients should be automatically referred to online patient education in the language of their choice. As a result, PHR systems will likely become lightweight content management systems, automating the delivery of targeted health content.

Eventually, meaningful use will begin to require EHR systems to accept uploads. Patient-generated data will likely first be manually or automatically uploaded into a PHR system, and then accepted into the EHR system. Of course, this is a further mandate for communication infrastructures like Direct and IHE. Indivo-style PHR platforms are already working on accepting and managing patient-generated data, but the PHRs that come tethered with EHR systems will likely have minimal capacity to accept it. Patient-generated data is at best vaguely defined. Communities like the quantters and e-patients will very likely prove the crucial value of very new and different forms of patient-generated data at a far faster pace than standards bodies will sort out how EHR systems should treat such data. Still, even with a lag, accepting patient-generated data even for simple record correction or commentary will be a huge technical step forward.

CHAPTER 7

Human Error

A lot of the drive toward IT in healthcare aims at eliminating human error from critical processes. This includes activities such as prescribing medications and properly handling complex treatment for chronic conditions. However, the introduction of new technologies presents its own risks that can in some cases be equally problematic with the human errors they reduce. Let's now take a look at common human errors, technological solutions, and the new risks they introduce.

In the context of meaningful use, the myopic focus on incentive payments has glossed over the fact that the prevention of medical errors is one of the core goals that drove its creation. The healthcare industry as a whole, perhaps naturally, put all its attention on the incentive payment process, but it is important to think about what the ultimate goals of the guidelines are. Many of them parrot the conclusions of several studies that focused on preventable medical errors and their resolutions. The recommended process for e-prescribing derives from the conclusions of a study mentioned in Chapter 1 and that we will focus on in more detail shortly, "To Err Is Human." Many more of the clinical guidelines come from several studies that found inconsistency and forgetfulness in the treatment of diabetes and hypertension, which involve complex and long-term treatments. Finally the auditing and historical action tracking guidelines allow for an honest and thorough accounting of mistakes when they inevitably occur. Although there is much academic literature on these topics, we feel a better introduction can be made through a series of illustrative anecdotes regarding unforeseen consequences and creative solutions.

The Extent of Error

Complex systems like healthcare are remarkably susceptible to simple mistakes, especially those made by the human elements of the process. The stakes couldn't be higher, as often a patient's life really does hang in the balance. From various studies and sources it becomes clear that even under the most conservative estimates, more than 40,000 patients a year die as a result of a preventable medical error. Some less conservative estimates put the number as high as 210,000 deaths per year. To put those numbers in perspective, motor vehicle accidents account for nearly 70,000 fatalities per year. When you think about the mind share and media attention paid to automotive accidents, it seems strangely disproportionate to the relatively little attention paid to the issue of medical errors.

A dated but still remarkably relevant study, especially in a slow-to-change industry such as healthcare, was conducted in the late 1990s. It is known by the iconic title "To Err Is Human," and it shocked readers by exposing a substantially higher level of human error than had been generally perceived at the time. Several further studies continued to validate and even extend the results found. The stand-out problem areas found by the study related to prescriptions and medication interactions.

The tangible action in response was the advent of several government and private initiatives to study in detail and begin to test implementations of methods to reduce the occurrence of errors. The majority of the methods to reduce errors ultimately involved technological changes and systems. After much review and distillation, those have become many of the core requirements of meaningful use. Unfortunately those methods to reduce errors have seen only modest adoption to date.

It should not come as a surprise when we delve in and look at the causes of error. They're the same as the errors we run into on an almost daily basis as we purchase goods at stores, interact with our families, and collaborate with others at work or in school. The vectors of error center on the legibility of handwritten text, transposition of characters and digits, imprecision in basic math, and inattentiveness to similar but distinct names and actions.

Those kinds of mistakes are just as common and possibly more common in a medical environment, where practitioners often operate under high stress and little sleep. Fortunately, computerized systems are very good at addressing all of those vectors, except for the issues where it is easy for a user to confuse similar entries. This is often true when there are many items having similar but slightly different names. Drug names are an example where computer interfaces can introduce confusion that might not exist in the paper world. For example, Celebrex and Celexa can be confused easily when making a selection from a drop-down list or autocomplete selection. Although fundamental research is underway in healthcare on these issues, general usability research going back to the dawn of modern computing uncovers these problems in other fields.

In many circles, including those who gave input to designing the meaningful use criteria, computerized systems are viewed as a panacea to eliminating medical error. Unfortunately we are beginning to see that computerized systems are only a tool to assist in reducing errors, and in all too many scenarios they introduce additional complexity that shifts errors to other areas and personnel rather than actually reducing them.

To understand medical error, it is a good idea to delve into some real-world examples that illustrate the types of mistakes and dangers faced by the field. These examples also illustrate that no matter what the pedigree of the provider or facility, all humans are equally susceptible to these types of mistakes. We will review a couple of specific cases that are representative of the types of errors most likely to occur, how meaningful use criteria affect those scenarios, and what new vectors are created by the system that fulfill meaningful use adoption.

Before diving into the examples of medical error that we have selected here, which look at primarily provider and technological errors, it is worthwhile to make a brief comment about patient opportunities for preventing errors. Without a doubt, the best defense patients have to prevent medical error is their own attention to their treatment and needs. In some cases, that patients might need a relative or other caregiver to act in their interest. Having an independent, watchful, and vocal party is the vital factor, whether it is the patient or someone close to them. In many cases, patients defer judgment to the "process" of healthcare without paying detailed attention to their treatment and the procedures being recommended and performed on them. In some cases this is a necessary result of their disability from illness, but in many others it is a cultural element based on the perceived roles of patient and caregiver. As a fundamentally human process, the healthcare system is often short on the individual focus on individual patients and cases that is required to prevent mistakes.

Dangerous Dosing

Cedars-Sinai Hospital in Los Angeles is a widely respected facility, considered by many to be a pinnacle of modern and effective care on the world stage. They attract top-tier talent from the world's leading medical schools. Irrespective of that lofty reputation, they made a widely publicized and unfortunately all too common error in 2007 that has been a known vector for error for nearly 10 years. We make a point here of identifying the facility as responsible for the error rather than just the individuals involved. This is not a legal distinction. We aren't trying to place legal blame or answer more complex questions about who is financially and ethically responsible for the mistakes we'll discuss here, but we do feel strongly that the responsibility to prevent these mistakes is the responsibility of the facility and not something that could be adequately addressed by just the individuals directly involved. It is also very unfortunate that among the 15 (not a typo) times the error was made in roughly 24 hours, only the case of a celebrity really caught national attention.

Dennis Quaid, a well-known actor, went with his wife and their infant twin daughters to Cedars-Sinai in 2007 to follow up on medical complications just a few weeks after their surrogate birth. Both twins were almost killed due to improper dosing of a medication called Heparin. Thirteen other infants received the same improper dosing.

Briefly put, Heparin is an anticlotting agent. It stops blood from forming clots in order to keep it flowing without forming obstructions. That might not sound like a good thing, but Heparin is used very widely. It keeps donated blood from clotting into untransfusable masses, it helps manage complex surgeries where patients on the operating table need areas to clot and other areas to flow freely, and it is used routinely in smaller doses to all patients receiving IVs and many other kinds of procedures that penetrate the skin.

In the cluster of cases we're talking about here, patients received Heparin with a strength of 10,000 units per milliliter instead of the correct strength of 10 units per milliliter. The only visual difference was three small zeros on the small vial. In mathematical terms, three zeros is a humongous difference but with respect to human error, reading a 10 from a 10,000 is a pretty simple and easily made mistake.

What nearly killed the Quaid twins and the 13 others was portrayed in the media as a "grossly negligent" medical error and an unusual, isolated incident. It was characterized as a systemic failure of existing and otherwise proper policies and procedures. Based on our own experience and our own analysis, that picture is not very accurate. Similar errors are made by most of us several times a week and could be made at any time in many settings. A world-class hospital is no different than a corner store when it comes to human error. The package of the drug vial was misread, that's all. Ever go to the store and mean to get the low-fat cottage cheese and accidentally get the full-fat kind? That's the fundamental error made in this case.

Certainly, we as patients have a right to expect a higher standard from medical facilities than we do from ourselves at the corner store. But this type of error and even this exact error has occurred thousands of times in the preceding 10 years. So why wasn't it prevented at Cedars-Sinai? In terms of process design there were several checks and balances that were in place that should have caught this type of error.

Almost all aspects of health care do in fact have defined procedures for ensuring accuracy and safety. In the case of Heparin and all medication administration, there is a policy known as the five rights that, when practiced correctly, would have eliminated this error. It defines that medication administration should only occur when five things are confirmed as being correct: the right patient, the right time, the right dose, the right means of administration (medically called the *route*) and finally the right medication. Many workflows will involve checking the five rights more than once or by different personnel.

Cedars-Sinai did not follow the five rights policy, and the same physician who selected the dose failed to properly vet the crucial details. What failed went beyond that particular instance, at that particular facility and occurs systemically as evidenced by the number of the cases where exactly the same Heparin misdosing has occurred. There is currently a lawsuit in progress against the manufacturer of Heparin with respect to its labeling. Some amount of responsibility might lie in improving that labeling, but we feel it is secondary to the core issue of proper process control.

However reasonableness our expectations, they fall short of reality. The tricky thing about controlling errors is that any process designed to prevent them can itself fall victim to an error. If a given activity is repeated enough times even very small probabilities of mistakes become unreasonably frequent when lives are at stake.

Let's say for example that a medication administration process encompassing all its checks and balances is 99.99% accurate. To a lay person that probably sounds pretty good. What that means in practice, however, is that a facility on the scale of Cedars-Sinai, with more than 400,000 medication administration events per year, would still have a lot of errors. That level of accuracy, which sounded good a moment ago, results in errors 40 times a year. Not all of those mistakes would result in death or even an adverse event at all, but when looking at the stakes involved it might still be an unacceptably high frequency for most observers and patients.

Having said that about the 99.99% accuracy level, we have to let you know that the real picture is much, much worse. Many basic studies of human reliability show that in repetitive processes it is unusual for us, even under ideal circumstances, to be accurate more than 99.98% of the time. Under high stress that falls to only 92% of the time. Those results are extremely sobering when considered At the medical context. In the scale we spoke about a moment ago it would mean between 80 and 32,000 mistaken doses per year.

A seminal error in health care history happened at the Dana Farber Cancer Institute in 1994 that also relates to medication dosing. This dosing error involved chemotherapy medication and had a tragic and fatal result. A protocol description for an experimental treatment for several patients was ambiguous, "cyclophosphamide dose 4 grams/square meter (of body surface area) over 4 days." The doctor ordering the medication assumed that meant 4 grams each day. But the protocol had been intended to mean 4 grams total over 4 days. One patient died, a couple were permanently harmed, and a few managed to recover after severe reactions.

That led Dana Farber to a 10-year obsessive focus on safety, and they became an early adopter of computerized systems to assist in improving safety. The net results of that effort are both positive and promising, but the scale of the effort is daunting. A world leading institution spent $11 million over 10 years on concerted efforts involving people and process, and became much safer. However, they still made 28 self-reported errors from 1997 to 2003 over a range of roughly 800,000 medication events. That means they were correct a visually impressive 99.999965% of the time. We leave it to the reader to ponder whether that is enough and what level of accuracy can be reached by a less well-funded organization with significantly greater challenges than Dana Farber.

A solution to the problem begins with basic education about the limitations of human processes, and in many cases this makes an excellent background on which to build a comprehensive meaningful use implementation. Although meaningful use involves computerized systems, the quest to eliminate error is absolutely not technology for technology's sake, like many other technological fads in healthcare.

In our opinion the ultimate failure in the Dana Farber case and in the majority of Heparin misdoses is one of culture and accountability. Technology played a role in the errors, but was just one tool in a vast workflow. If the driver of a car tailgates another car and applies the brakes too late to prevent a rear-end collision we don't include the vehicle in assessing accountability. There is plenty of information available in many of the studies and reports done after the fact. That said, stuck with paper processes and the lack of an interactive framework, it is possible at times for the error rate to sneak upward due to human tendencies. Computerized systems for meaningful use go a long way toward providing that rigid and repeatable framework that encourages humans to follow proper procedures 100% of the time.

In reducing the likelihood of dosing errors, meaningful use provides a strong process framework. That framework encompasses proper patient identification, proper medication selection, proper dosing selection (with the possibility for improper dosing floors and ceilings), proper method of administration, and proper scheduling of medications. Many meaningful use systems also support tools that might automate the physical selection of the correct drug (such as a barcode scan). The rigidity of those determinations in the computerized system contrasts with the inconsistent application of the five rights in the paper world that played a role in the Heparin dosing errors we considered a moment ago.

Rigidity is both the benefit and frustration produced by meaningful use systems. They are inflexible, requiring rigid adherence to a specific set of steps each and every time an action is performed. That is the opposite of our experience and expectations with human processes and not without its own problems, which we discuss later in this chapter as well as Chapter 4.

The undercurrents of meaningful use are very strongly based on defining and requiring a consistent, accurate, and safe workflow. Focusing purely on technological tools will miss the primary benefit and challenge of implementing meaningful use properly. To faithfully bring its spirit to life, compliance requires a top to bottom analysis of your facility's workflow and where to effectuate change that brings nonsystemic and ad-hoc processes into a consistent mold. The beneficial side effect of this focus on workflow consistency is substantially improved safety.

Discontents of Computerization

Technology offers a few easy solutions to the problems of human error. The type of repetitive, laborious steps that are often the root of human error are extremely well suited to the machine precision and efficiency of computerized systems. The real challenge is understanding that for all the paths to error technology solves, it introduces a variety of new and potentially even more dangerous paths. It is a vital precept that computerized systems must never be a substitute for human analysis, review and judgment, they are only a supplement to those things.

Computerized systems, including those certified for meaningful use, suffer from a significant flaw found in all computers: they operate only in the method they were programmed and on the data they are provided. In the realm of computer-generated error, let's now take a look at a very tragic one, albeit one unrelated to meaningful use.

Medical scans provide a sobering case of how technology can play a role in creating errors. Health care has a fairly long history of using radiation and radiological systems for many kinds of scans and imaging. These nuclear systems employ the same physics that might be found in a power plant or a bomb, but harnessed for clinical treatment or diagnosis. Many scans, including cat scans (CTs) and X-Rays, involve nuclear radiation in one form or another. The same kind of radiation that can cause radiation sickness, cancer, and deaths (as we have seen around the Japanese Fukoshima Reactor meltdowns) has many utilitarian purposes in medicine. Unfortunately, in the past 10 years, the machines used to deploy the radiation in healthcare have suffered from an uncomfortably high rate of error. Those errors have resulted in radiation overdoses that caused permanent disability and patient deaths.

One of the more prevalent series of cases involves software that manages linear accelerator equipment. That is another medical tool that utilizes radiation for the treatment of certain illnesses. In a scenario familiar to all of us who use desktop or laptop computers, the software was prone to freezing and crashing. In some cases, a system crash would reset the parameters that had been set for a particular patient scan to their default settings. This led to hundreds of cases where patients received enormous overdoses of radiation.

The operators of the system were certainly aware of the freezing and crashing, but they failed to understand the implications. In computerized systems, as this example shows, proper defaults and failsafes are a crucial element in protecting patients. The technicians in this case were well trained, but they were not computer scientists. They did not have the background with software to understand how the system might behave after it crashed and whether problematic defaults might be re-enabled after the technician had adjusted them one time at the beginning.

No physical failsafe, such as independent radiation measures for checking the calibration on each scan was available or even conceived of. Everyone involved blindly trusted the system. The FDA had approved the software, the vendors of the equipment involved had tested it, but a combination of updates to the underlying operating system, practices of hospital IT, and a poor understanding of computerized systems led to the confluence of events that caused the errors. Again, proper practices of the "5 rights" vein combined with proper use of computerized systems would have prevented the errors, and in hindsight the situation seems outrageous. Many patients might feel uncomfortable challenging a scene where the scanning system has crashed multiple times, but it could have certainly been a point of discussion at the very least. Unfortunately, the patients were not even informed that the system crashed and needed to be restarted.

The heart of the problem in the case we just reviewed is one of integrated systems. Each piece appeared to work reliably in isolation, but the combination introduced new vectors for problems. Over periods of time, those vectors expanded until the overall lack of reliability results in tragic consequences. Unfortunately, at this point meaningful use does not offer comment or support with respect to the overall system integration at a site. It is up to your organization to take responsibility for using the meaningful use certified system in a way that improves safety.

Process Errors and Organizational Change

So we have now looked at a purely human type of error and an integrated systems error. Now we will look at a fundamentally process-related type of error, wrong side surgeries. All of us have made this kind of error, mixing up left and right, or top and bottom, at one point or another, but it has far more serious consequences in healthcare. Although hard to properly count across all procedures, some studies show that this happens approximately 3,000 times per year. Roughly 20 million surgeries are done each year, so a basic rule of thumb shows that surgeries operate on the correct side 99.99985% of the time. Again, as we start out that looks like an impressive level of accuracy, but when we keep stacking other types of errors together including dosing and systems errors we reviewed, the inaccuracies add up to a serious health care crisis.

Wrong side surgeries represent a particularly problematic type of error because in many cases a new problem will have been added on top of the existing one. This is a horrendous tragedy when a healthy kidney has been removed, leaving the diseased one in the patient. What could have been a somewhat straightforward and positive result becomes escalated in to a potentially lethal and arduous risk-prone consequence.

One disconcerting aspect of a wrong side surgery is that it typically involves the failure of more than one person who comes in contact with the patient. The other disconcerting aspect is that in a majority of cases, both the written and electronic presurgical records and orders reflect the proper side. Humans are fundamentally bad at mirrored positions, we have a likelihood of absentmindedly coming to different conclusions given the same information. How many of us, in a given day or week have said, "Your left or my left?" The thought of a surgical team asking the same question sends a shudder through most of us.

In the handoff between diagnosing a problem, determining a treatment, and finally conferring that information to the surgical team when the treatment involves surgery, there are a lot of opportunities for reversing positions of a problem. Contrary to what can often be found in medical literature, medical imaging often uses the literal "left" and "right" type terminology. Radiologists and highly skilled providers are more likely to use specific Latin-based terminology such as "medio-lateral axis." However that discounts the other 6 to 10 people with whom the patient might have had contact from the receptionist to various technicians. Many folks might dispute this claim, but more than two decades of collective experience by the authors at hundreds of facilities shows the lay speak is still very common. Typically, left and right in imaging, when looking at a computer screen or physical film, refer to the orientation you would see when facing the patient with their head oriented vertically toward the sky. In that scenario, the patient's "left" side (as the patient would describe it) is on the right side of the view. That is a recipe for confusion and error.

Problems can arise on several fronts with imaging. Many other departments use different terminology, and surgeons might again use different terminology than those other departments and imaging professionals. During the explanation process with the patient and in their consent paperwork, the lay-speak "left" and "right" might be used yet again. Combine all those people and all those opportunities for reversal, and one can see a large number of points for an error to be introduced. In our own experience, we have seen an uncomfortable number of times that a wrong side error occurred, to be resolved accidentally but fortunately by a second wrong side error on the same patient. For the most part, we suspect cases like those go either unnoticed or unreported.

The solution to wrong side surgeries can be difficult to resolve using computerized systems due to the fundamental human tendencies we have already identified. The solution involves defining a culture and process that consistently describes the procedures and patients in a similar way and using means that cannot be mirrored or reversed. In practice, this all requires significant training, changes to entrenched behaviors, and consensus building that does not come easily to territorial departments. The Joint Commission on Accreditation of Healthcare Organizations (JCAHO), which is responsible for accrediting hospital operations, fostered the "Universal Protocol For Preventing Wrong Site, Wrong Procedure, Wrong Person Surgery" in 2003. But at this time of writing, 2011, the number of wrong side surgeries has not been dramatically reduced. Some other competing protocols exist as well, but the issue has clearly been adoption and application rather than the means themselves.

The "wrong side" problem is perhaps the most relevant in understanding the limitations that meaningful use adoption will encounter in the quest to fundamentally eliminate preventable medical errors. With respect to wrong side surgery, it is known what the problem is, what causes it, and what tools can eliminate it, yet the errors are still being made. Meaningful use is in a similar boat. When properly employed it has enormous potential to increase patient safety, but that bit about "properly employed" is a very steep hill to climb.

The lesson to take away from this chapter is what we call the *triangle of errors*, which can be thought of briefly as human error, system error, and process error. Meaningful use cannot fundamentally stop humans from intending one thing and accidentally doing another, but it can address system errors and process errors that reduce the impact of human mistakes. On the downside, meaningful use also introduces many new opportunities for unanticipated problems that would otherwise not be present in a paper system. As a general rule, medical professionals are not technologists and do not have a good fundamental understanding of computers and computerized systems, which can exacerbate problems.

We saw with the nuclear medicine software how poorly chosen defaults combined with technicians' poor understanding of computer systems and how machines could accidentally reset, resulting in needless patient deaths. By comparison, such single-purpose machines are much more simplistic than the myriad of needs addressed by meaningful use certified systems, so an extraordinary degree of care needs to be taken as meaningful use is rolled out. However, the real-world cases of error we discussed here are powerful and convincing evidence that advocates of meaningful use can cite to make organizations take notice and reassess previously held assumptions about safety.

Deep Medical Errors and EHR Solutions

As a final example, we can review a scenario relating to human error by both providers and patients. This example focuses on the risks caused by cumulative dosing in nuclear medicine and is both very current and somewhat controversial. We have talked about how improperly programmed CT scans resulted in patient deaths, but now we will discuss the risks and errors that might occur even with properly programmed and calibrated CT scans in a proper process.

A CT scan is an invaluable diagnostic tool, but one that uses potentially dangerous radiation to generate its noninvasive image. The problem that is beginning to raise concerns is that radiation exposure is cumulative over your lifetime. Every additional X-ray or CT scan you have slightly increases the likelihood of developing cancer or other complications.

An overly simple way of explaining the challenges presented from cumulative dosing is to imagine a patient visiting the ER because she suffered a moderate head injury, such as commonly occurs from an accidental kick at a soccer match. To rule out potential risks from concussion and other complications, such as bleeding in the brain, CT scans are commonly done. The current point of controversy arises when no acute problem is found. That might be a relief to the patient on that day, but the radiation from those scans might cause a fatal cancer 10 years later. Medically speaking, it would have been a better practice to take a wait-and-see approach with the patient and her symptoms. But that potentially raises liability concerns for the provider and is often disconcerting to patients with a typically "more is better" attitude.

The medical error involves a failure to carefully and thoughtfully understand a patient's history of exposure to radiation from historical scans or other sources. Naturally, current U.S. practice does not provide such a comprehensive, life-long history when the patient arrives at the emergency room. Second, there is the potential for error when depending too much on the use of scans for reasons of cost, expedience, and liability. Although a wait-and see-approach, where the patient can return to the hospital for a scan if additional symptoms or risk factors present themselves, might be less comforting to the patient and is somewhat nonintuitive, this is a case where refraining from a diagnostic procedure results in a better long-term outcome for the patient.

Patients themselves contribute to this error in two ways: first by pursuing a more-is-always-better approach to their treatment and diagnosis and second by failing to properly understand and communicate their history of radiological exposure from imaging and other sources.

When first introduced to oncology, the diagnosis and treatment of cancer, one author of this book was quite surprised to learn about the frequent use of CT scans to examine tumors. Evidence is beginning to emerge that overutilization of radiological scans permits an oncologist to "cure" a current cancer only to cause a future one. This is a case of poor medical judgment that is very different from the kinds of errors we have examined so far in this chapter. It is important to state that the element of error is subtle but presents very dangerous long-term consequences for patients, and that the error has been almost completely ignored because of its long time frame.

EHRs offer a wonderful opportunity to mitigate this type of subtle, long-term risk and prevent error because they can deliver to providers the information they need to properly manage risks in each specific patient situation. The interoperability guidelines in meaningful use also provide an excellent foundation for fostering the efficient sharing of record information that is contextual to preventing cumulative overexposure. Across-the-board use of electronic records, together with the secure data exchange networks described elsewhere in this book, could allow every provider in an emergency situation to review the patient's radiation history in a time frame consistent with the decision the provider and patient need to make.

Errors Caused by Human-Computer Mismatch

You don't know what you don't know; that's the most common problem of moving to computerized EHR systems. If users do not fully comprehend the operation of the window they are looking at on the computer, a new potential vector for errors is introduced. Filters, pagination mechanisms, and basic screen or window behaviors can create problem scenarios where users might think they are seeing all available information, but in fact are seeing only a subset. They can then make erroneous medical decisions because of incomplete information.

At a customer of ClearHealth, we encountered a situation where a specific department of an organization was not seeing the abnormal flags on electronic lab results. Their job, which they were doing as well as they could given their level of knowledge, was to manually review each lab result on the screen and determine whether the result was within a normal range. They consistently failed to notice that the lab had flagged results as abnormal. Complicating matters, the staff didn't even know that the system was automatically showing abnormal flags for lab results. Fortunately no patients were harmed as a result, but it certainly added a lot of work for the practice and created high potential for making mistakes.

What caused this fundamental problem? The department had older monitors running at an unusual resolution, which caused the right side of the screen to be clipped, hiding the abnormal flag column. In training, users had been shown that in general, moving the mouse to a particular area scrolled the screen. But as staff turnover occurred, that knowledge was slowly lost. They didn't know what they didn't know until some users reviewed our online training videos and asked why they did not have the abnormal column feature enabled.

The lesson is to consider having homogeneous equipment for high risk areas and make sure it is tested thoroughly. Different operation system versions, resolutions, and monitors have caused a lot of similar problems that we have witnessed or heard about anecdotally in the time we have been implementing EHRs.

Across many views in the electronic world, more data is available than can be presented on screen. There are two primary mechanisms to address this: scrolling and pagination. It is very important that users understand those concepts. Otherwise, they can miss out on a lot of information and potentially make erroneous decisions based on incomplete information. Pagination in particular can be tricky for users with average or lower computer proficiency. Often it can be difficult to understand user issues like this without viewing actual users in their actual setting using the system. A good training program will include real-world observation as its final step before deployment, and from time to time as the system continues to be used.

Finally, the newest problem introduced by meaningful use compliant EHR systems is known as alert fatigue. This is the tendency of humans to make mistakes in commonly repeated and consistent operations involving on-screen prompts. How many of us have trained our brains to click OK on the popup that appears every time we install a new program? The same instinct can kick in when a computer prompts repeatedly with warnings or alerts. The danger level of those alerts is that they are visually homogeneous and vary only through small icons or sometimes color. If users receive too many erroneous or useless notices in a popup format, they can be conditioned to plow through them and miss an important prompt when it does appear, perhaps regarding something such as a potentially lethal medication interaction.

This type of error was discussed at length during the meaningful use comment process and most vendors have made strong efforts to keep erroneous popups to a minimum. Again though, you need to make sure your organization sets proper defaults unique to your workflow. A crucial alert for a podiatry practice might be a useless notification for an internal medicine department.

Best Practices

Having covered errors in this chapter, we have a few specific pieces of advice that relate to your meaningful use implementation and the steps you can take to reduce or eliminate errors at your practice. Conveniently, those steps also provide us an excellent opportunity to weave in a few general-purpose points for your implementation as well.

Survey and provide training regarding basic computer skills.
     I can count on one hand the number of facilities who said their staff had above average computer skills and whose staff actually did. More than 50% of users at the rest of sites self-reported as average or below average on an anonymous survey.

By basic computer skills we are referring to a pyramid of proficiencies, starting with the physical skills of typing and using a mouse. Above that foundation is a conceptual understanding of what a computer consists of, what an operating system and application software are, short-term storage of data, and long-term storage of data. Above that come the mechanics of using the operating system and application software, starting and stopping programs, controlling windows, window focus, and how software interacts with a network, including the Internet and email. We've seen that fewer than 50% of medical professionals posses that pyramid of basic skills at the level needed to successfully use a meaningful use compliant EHR.

Study carefully the history of errors, both reported and unreported, that your facility has made.

Larger facilities almost always have ongoing policies and procedures to perform this type of analysis, but it is often absent at medium and smaller organizations. It can be a very uncomfortable area of discussion, but medicine has several specific carve-outs in the law to conduct this type of review without incurring liability. Consult your organization's legal representation, but make sure to do this type of review in some capacity.

Create workflow diagrams that describe the on-the-ground, real-world process for patient workflows.

It is not necessary to cover every conceivable scenario at your facility, but getting all departments to agree on common use cases regarding how a patient traverses a facility is always an illuminating process for the parties involved. Rarely do most departments' impressions of their operations match the reality on the ground. Most of the time, the perception and reality differ wildly. Improving that understanding and communication has a direct correlation to efficiency and accuracy in patient care.

Do not use generic training materials. Create organizationally specific training programs in coordination with your vendors.

Most vendors provide a generic, one-size-fits-all training program and training materials. Inevitably, your real-world needs will result in some configurations in the software that differ from the generic materials. As staff changes over time, workflow problems and mistakes will arise because the training materials differ from the on-the-ground workflow. This is the ideal environment for medical errors to be introduced into an otherwise safely operating organization.

Review comprehensively the defaults of your chosen system and whether they present any danger to patients, especially in unusual circumstances.

I cannot think of a system that ships with defaults appropriate for all cases. Systems cannot be one size fits all. Carefully and comprehensively review the default state of all important areas and functions and how they can be triggered to reset. Document things that require changing and challenge some of your staff to invent scenarios that are infrequent or can present unexpected challenges. Use those eccentric scenarios to test your system and identify potentially problematic areas.

Conduct periodic retraining of staff and process audits.

EHR systems offer an enormous number of features and there can be a steep learning curve for many users moving from long-entrenched paper processes to computerized systems. Some selective retraining on an annual basis can greatly help users as they can review less used features in a more contemporary and personal context. They can also identify things that are the so-called unknown unknowns, things they weren't aware they did not know.

IT personnel must be told about the seriousness of care-related IT systems versus noncare systems.

It is up to the IT department to carefully manage change and determine risks as updates, upgrades, and versions evolve. It is crucial that the people responsible for those decisions weigh those factors differently in the context of systems that are used to treat patients. This can be very frustrating, but patient safety has to take a priority over other aspects of IT management.

Getting an IT department to provide a different type of support or level of thinking about a specific system can be daunting, but in this case it rarely requires significant changes to policy. It just entails better, more detailed, and more frequent communication about changes. It is also very important to create upgrade processes that allow for reversal of changes, or to roll out changes incrementally so you can identify problems before they affect all providers and patients at once.

In conclusion, we assert that patient safety does not improve merely by changing to computerized systems. It is improved only when three distinct and fundamental areas of the practice are addressed simultaneously: the triangle of human, system, and process errors. You need to create consistent processes that human actors use as a basis for operations, and to control and test errors that can occur via the computerized system. Evaluate your practice as a whole and be careful of a myopia that sees only your most common situations or most widely trafficked departments.

CHAPTER 8

Meaningful Use Overview

What actually is meaningful use? Even though the term arises whenever the current U.S. healthcare system is under discussion, we find very few people who are actually familiar with the specifics of each guideline and requirement. A little background first is important.

Many people wrongly believe that meaningful use was part of the healthcare legislation passed by Congress in 2010. In fact, it was part of the economic stimulus passed more than a year before, the American Reinvestment Recovery Act (ARRA). That bill set aside $20 billion for incentives to encourage medical practices and hospitals to use new technologies such as EHRs—but in specific and accountable ways that are denoted by the term *meaningful use*. These uses include gathering clear statistics on patient illnesses, improving interaction with patients and others using the Internet, and utilizing accuracy and error control systems such as ePrescribing.

As with many government regulations, the ARRA offers a problematic amount to sort through. We have digested and analyzed the 5,000+ pages of legislation and rule-making by HHS, ONC, and CMS and created this concise interactive guide to help you understand the specific criteria that can make you meaningful use compliant and eligible to receive the current incentive payments. The guidelines are very different depending on whether you are part of an outpatient practice (ambulatory) or a hospital facility (inpatients). We list the outpatient guidelines first, followed by inpatient facilities.

Meaningful use objectives are broken down into two distinct groups for determining Stage 1 (the current year) compliance: a core set of objectives and a menu set. A meaningful user must satisfy all objectives under the core set, and 5 of the 10 menu set objectives. In the list that follows, the "Criteria" sections define the meaningful use objectives, and the "Measure" sections define the reporting threshold that must be met to demonstrate meaningful use for the associated objective.

Outpatient Guidelines and Requirements

All of the measures in the core set are required for meaningful use compliance.

Because of the fluid nature of the meaningful use requirements and the ongoing rule-making, it is important to check with the registration website (*http://www.cms.gov/EHRIncentivePrograms/20_RegistrationandAttestation.asp*) for the latest information:

Guideline #1

> *Computerized Provider Order Entry (CPOE)*
>> Use of CPOE for medication orders directly entered by any licensed healthcare professional who can enter orders into the medical record per state, local, and professional guidelines. This guideline covers ePrescribing as well as the recording of medications that are dispensed and administered within the facility.

> *Measure*
>> More than 30% of unique patients seen by the eligible provider (eligible hospital's or critical access hospital's [CAH] inpatient or emergency department), who have at least one medication in their medication list, have at least one medication order entered using CPOE.

Guideline #2

> *Drug Allergy Checking*
>> Implement drug-drug and drug-allergy interaction checks. Typically this guideline involves both drug-to-allergy and drug-to-drug contraindications, although there is flexibility in the guidelines text in this regard.

> *Guideline #2 Measure*
>> The eligible hospital's or CAH's inpatient or emergency department has enabled this functionality for the entire EHR reporting period.

Guideline #3

> *ePrescribing (eRx)*
>> Generate and transmit permissible prescriptions electronically (eRx). As a practical matter, at the time of this writing, only Surescripts is recognized as a valid bureau for the transmission of electronic prescriptions to pharmacies for outpatient facilities, although the guideline itself does not mention Surescripts by name.

> *Measure*
>> More than 40% of all permissible prescriptions written by the eligible provider (eligible hospital's or CAH's inpatient or emergency department) are transmitted electronically using certified EHR technology.

Guideline #4

Record Demographics

These include preferred language, gender, race, ethnicity, and date of birth. Some of that data is already tracked by most facilities, but preferred language, race, and ethnicity are new demographics to many lines of care.

Measure

More than 50% of all unique patients seen by the eligible provider (eligible hospital's or CAH's inpatient or emergency department) have demographics recorded as structured data.

Guideline #5

Problem List

Maintain an up-to-date problem list of current and active diagnoses.

Measure

More than 80% of all unique patients seen by the eligible provider (eligible hospital's or CAH's inpatient or emergency department) have at least one entry or an indication, recorded as structured data, that no problems are known for the patient. Structured data here refers to the ability to report distinctly on individual problems by code. A clinical note recorded during a patient-provider interaction is insufficient to comply with this guideline.

Guideline #6

Medication List

Maintain an active medication list detailing medications the patient is actively taking that are prescribed by the provider's facility or reported by the patient. Again, this guidelines requires data on each individual medication and cannot be complied with using only text clinical notes.

Measure

More than 80% of all unique patients seen by the eligible provider (eligible hospital's or CAH's inpatient or emergency department) have at least one entry (or an indication that the patient is not currently prescribed any medication), recorded as structured data.

Guideline #7

Allergy List

Maintain an active medication allergy list that tracks medication allergies, at a minimum. All meaningful use certified systems to date also permit tracking of environmental, food, and other miscellaneous allergies as well as medications.

Measure

More than 80% of all unique patients seen by the eligible provider (eligible hospital's or CAH's inpatient or emergency department) have at least one entry (or an indication that the patient has no known medication allergies) recorded as structured data.

Guideline #8

Vital Signs

Record patient vitals as part of typical workflow. Vital signs include taking height, weight, and blood pressure, calculating and displaying body mass index (BMI), and plotting and displaying growth charts for children 2 to 20 years old including BMI. This measure will be a significant workflow change for many types of facilities not accustomed to tracking vital statistics with this level of detail on each visit. A few select exemptions apply; please check CMS advisories for more information. The reasoning for this measure, even in lines of care where the necessity for vitals might not be immediately apparent, is that vital statistics provide a solid evidentiary base for earlier prevention of the most problematic chronic diseases, and each interaction with a provider of any specialty is a good opportunity for this basic prevention step.

Measure

For more than 50% of all unique patients age 2 and over seen by the eligible provider (eligible hospital's or CAH's inpatient or emergency department), record height, weight, and blood pressure as structured data.

Guideline #9

Smoking Status

Record smoking status for patients 13 years old or older. Again, this guideline applies to all specialties, even those that have not historically tracked this information and even if it is not immediately obvious how it might be connected to their practices. Smoking-related illness remains a significant cause of adverse health, and any interaction with a medical provider of any kind is a good opportunity to help patients stop smoking or to create correlating data about all types of illness and smoking.

Measure

More than 50% of all unique patients 13 years old or older seen by the eligible provider (eligible hospital's or CAH's inpatient or emergency department) have smoking status recorded.

Guideline #10

Clinical Decision Support (CDS)

Implement one clinical decision support rule relevant to specialty or high clinical priority, along with the ability to track compliance for this rule. Clinical decision support remains the holy grail of EHRs in many circles. It is an advanced concept where the system can apply logical conditions to known data points and make recommendations or present evidentiary advisements about possible diagnosis, treatment, and outcomes for the patient. CDS is a radical jump toward consistent and systematized care, which is still rare in the United States today. CDS is expected to play a larger and larger role as guidelines continue to expand in future years. This guideline provides enormous flexibility in compliance and sets a low bar, requiring the provider to implement only a single CDS rule, no matter how simplistic. To a large extent, this guideline is an indicator and placeholder to introduce facilities to the concept.

Measure

Implement one clinical decision support rule.

Guideline #11

Report Clinical Quality Measures

Report ambulatory clinical quality measures to CMS or the states. This guideline takes the big step of actually demonstrating meaningful use compliance by submitting the summarized numbers, proving compliance with each guideline.

Measure

For 2011, provide aggregate numerator, denominator, and exclusions through attestation to the state or federal government through the web-based reporting system. The specific measures for outpatient facilities are itemized in the list that follows. Not all items have to be reported to be compliant. If you try to identify the heart of meaningful use, you could locate it in the ability to answer all of the questions in the list. These questions have been identified as critical by the leading agencies involved in funding and researching health and healthcare. Having a large, concise, and accurate pool of data regarding these issues is the best chance we have to improve patient outcomes in the system. Although the list is dense and filled with confusing terminology, it is important to spend a little time reviewing these questions and determining how your organization will need to change in order to be able to answer them.

NQF 0421
PQRI 128
Title: Adult Weight Screening and Follow-Up
Description: Percentage of patients aged 18 years and older whose BMI was calculated in the past six months or during the current visit and was documented in the medical record, in addition to which, if the most recent BMI is outside parameters, a follow-up plan is documented.

NQF 0013
Title: Hypertension: Blood Pressure Measurement
Description: Percentage of patient visits for patients aged 18 years and older with a diagnosis of hypertension who have been seen for at least two office visits, with blood pressure (BP) recorded.

NQF 0028
Title: Preventive Care and Screening Measure Pair: a. Tobacco Use Assessment, b. Tobacco Cessation Intervention
Description: a. Percentage of patients aged 18 years and older who have been seen for at least two office visits and who were queried about tobacco use one or more times within 24 months b. Percentage of patients aged 18

years and older identified as tobacco users within the past 24 months, who have been seen for at least two office visits, and who received cessation intervention.

NQF 0041
PQRI 110
Title: Preventive Care and Screening: Influenza Immunization for Patients ≥ 50 Years Old
Description: Percentage of patients aged 50 years and older who received an influenza immunization during the flu season (September through February).

NQF 0024
Title: Weight Assessment and Counseling for Children and Adolescents
Description: Percentage of patients 2 to 17 years of age who had an outpatient visit with a Primary Care Physician (PCP) or OB/GYN and who had evidence of BMI percentile documentation, counseling for nutrition, and counseling for physical activity during the measurement year.

NQF 0038
Title: Childhood Immunization Status
Description: Percentage of children 2 years of age who had four diphtheria, tetanus and acellular pertussis (DTaP); three polio (IPV), one measles, mumps and rubella (MMR); two H influenza type B (HiB); three hepatitis B (Hep B); one chicken pox (VZV); four pneumococcal conjugate (PCV); two hepatitis A (Hep A); two or three rotavirus (RV); and two influenza (flu) vaccines by their second birthday. The measure calculates a rate for each vaccine and nine separate combination rates.

NQF 0059
PQRI 1
Title: Diabetes: Hemoglobin A1c Poor Control
Description: Percentage of patients 18 to 75 years of age with diabetes (type 1 or type 2) who had hemoglobin A1c > 9.0%.

NQF 0064
PQRI 2
Title: Diabetes: Low Density Lipoprotein (LDL) Management and Control
Description: Percentage of patients 18 to 75 years of age with diabetes (type 1 or type 2) who had LDL-C <100 mg/dL).

NQF 0061
PQRI 3
Title: Diabetes: Blood Pressure Management
Description: Percentage of patients 18 to 75 years of age with diabetes (type 1 or type 2) who had blood pressure < 140/90 mmHg.

NQF 0081
PQRI 5
Title: Heart Failure (HF): Angiotensin-Converting Enzyme (ACE) Inhibitor or Angiotensin Receptor Blocker (ARB) Therapy for Left Ventricular Systolic Dysfunction (LVSD)
Description: Percentage of patients aged 18 years and older with a diagnosis of heart failure and LVSD (LVEF lt; 40%) who were prescribed ACE inhibitor or ARB therapy.

NQF 0070
PQRI 7
Title: Coronary Artery Disease (CAD): Beta-Blocker Therapy for CAD Patients with Prior Myocardial Infarction (MI)
Description: Percentage of patients aged 18 years and older with a diagnosis of CAD and prior MI who were prescribed beta-blocker therapy.

NQF 0043
PQRI 111
Title: Pneumonia Vaccination Status for Older Adults
Description: Percentage of patients 65 years of age and older who have ever received a pneumococcal vaccine.

NQF 0031
PQRI 112
Title: Breast Cancer Screening
Description: Percentage of women 40 to 69 years of age who had a mammogram to screen for breast cancer.

NQF 0034
PQRI 113
Title: Colorectal Cancer Screening
Description: Percentage of adults 50 to 75 years of age who had appropriate screening for colorectal cancer.

NQF 0067
PQRI 6
Title: Coronary Artery Disease (CAD): Oral Antiplatelet Therapy Prescribed for Patients with CAD
Description: Percentage of patients aged 18 years and older with a diagnosis of CAD who were prescribed oral antiplatelet therapy.

NQF 0083
PQRI 8
Title: Heart Failure (HF): Beta-Blocker Therapy for Left Ventricular Systolic Dysfunction (LVSD)

Description: Percentage of patients aged 18 years and older with a diagnosis of heart failure who also have LVSD (LVEF lt; 40%) and who were prescribed beta-blocker therapy.

NQF 0105
PQRI 9
Title: Anti-Depressant Medication Management: (a) Effective Acute Phase Treatment,(b)Effective Continuation Phase Treatment
Description: The percentage of patients 18 years of age and older who were diagnosed with a new episode of major depression, treated with antidepressant medication, and who remained on an antidepressant medication treatment.

NQF 0086
PQRI 12
Title: Primary Open Angle Glaucoma (POAG): Optic Nerve Evaluation
Description: Percentage of patients aged 18 years and older with a diagnosis of POAG who have been seen for at least two office visits who have an optic nerve head evaluation during one or more office visits within 12 months.

NQF 0088
PQRI 18
Title: Diabetic Retinopathy: Documentation of Presence or Absence of Macular Edema and Level of Severity of Retinopathy
Description: Percentage of patients aged 18 years and older with a diagnosis of diabetic retinopathy who had a dilated macular or fundus exam performed that included documentation of the level of severity of retinopathy and the presence or absence of macular edema during one or more office visits within 12 months.

NQF 0089
PQRI 19
Title: Diabetic Retinopathy: Communication with the Physician Managing Ongoing Diabetes Care
Description: Percentage of patients aged 18 years and older with a diagnosis of diabetic retinopathy who had a dilated macular or fundus exam performed with documented communication to the physician who manages the ongoing care of the patient with diabetes mellitus regarding the findings of the macular or fundus exam at least once within 12 months.

NQF 0047
PQRI 53
Title: Asthma Pharmacologic Therapy
Description: Percentage of patients aged 5 through 40 years with a diagnosis of mild, moderate, or severe persistent asthma who were prescribed

either the preferred long-term control medication (inhaled corticosteroid) or an acceptable alternative treatment.

NQF 0001
PQRI 64
Title: Asthma Assessment
Description: Percentage of patients aged 5 through 40 years with a diagnosis of asthma and who have been seen for at least two office visits, who were evaluated during at least one office visit within 12 months for the frequency (numeric) of daytime and nocturnal asthma symptoms.

NQF 0002
PQRI 66
Title: Appropriate Testing for Children with Pharyngitis
Description: Percentage of children 2 to 18 years of age who were diagnosed with pharyngitis, dispensed an antibiotic, and received a group A streptococcus (strep) test for the episode.

NQF 0387
PQRI 71
Title: Oncology Breast Cancer: Hormonal Therapy for Stage IC-IIIC Estrogen Receptor/Progesterone Receptor (ER/PR) Positive Breast Cancer
Description: Percentage of female patients aged 18 years and older with Stage IC through IIIC, ER or PR positive breast cancer who were prescribed tamoxifen or aromatase inhibitor (AI) during the 12-month reporting period.

NQF 0385
PQRI 72
Title: Oncology Colon Cancer: Chemotherapy for Stage III Colon Cancer Patients
Description: Percentage of patients aged 18 years and older with Stage IIIA through IIIC colon cancer who are referred for adjuvant chemotherapy, prescribed adjuvant chemotherapy, or have previously received adjuvant chemotherapy within the 12-month reporting period.

NQF 0389
PQRI 102
Title: Prostate Cancer: Avoidance of Overuse of Bone Scan for Staging Low-Risk Prostate Cancer Patients
Description: Percentage of patients, regardless of age, with a diagnosis of prostate cancer at low risk of recurrence receiving interstitial prostate brachytherapy, OR external beam radiotherapy to the prostate, OR radical prostatectomy, OR cryotherapy who did not have a bone scan performed at any time since diagnosis of prostate cancer.

NQF 0027

PQRI 115

Title: Smoking and Tobacco Use Cessation, Medical Assistance: a. Advising Smokers and Tobacco Users to Quit, b. Discussing Smoking and Tobacco Use Cessation Medications, c. Discussing Smoking and Tobacco Use Cessation Strategies

Description: Percentage of patients 18 years of age and older who were current smokers or tobacco users, who were seen by a practitioner during the measurement year, and who received advice to quit smoking or tobacco use or whose practitioner recommended or discussed smoking or tobacco use cessation medications, methods, or strategies.

NQF 0055
PQRI 117

Title: Diabetes: Eye Exam

Description: Percentage of patients 18 to 75 years of age with diabetes (type 1 or type 2) who had a retinal or dilated eye exam or a negative retinal exam (no evidence of retinopathy) by an eye care professional.

NQF 0062
PQRI 119

Title: Diabetes: Urine Screening

Description: Percentage of patients 18 to 75 years of age with diabetes (type 1 or type 2) who had a nephropathy screening test or evidence of nephropathy.

NQF 0056
PQRI 163

Title: Diabetes: Foot Exam

Description: The percentage of patients aged 18 to 75 years with diabetes (type 1 or type 2) who had a foot exam (visual inspection, sensory exam with monofilament, or pulse exam).

NQF 0074
PQRI 197

Title: Coronary Artery Disease (CAD): Drug Therapy for Lowering LDL Cholesterol

Description: Percentage of patients aged 18 years and older with a diagnosis of CAD who were prescribed a lipid-lowering therapy (based on current ACC/AHA guidelines).

NQF 0084
PQRI 200

Title: Heart Failure (HF): Warfarin Therapy Patients with Atrial Fibrillation

Description: Percentage of all patients aged 18 years and older with a diagnosis of heart failure and paroxysmal or chronic atrial fibrillation who were prescribed warfarin therapy.

NQF 0073
PQRI 201
Title: Ischemic Vascular Disease (IVD): Blood Pressure Management
Description: Percentage of patients 18 years of age and older who were discharged alive for acute myocardial infarction (AMI), coronary artery bypass graft (CABG), or percutaneous transluminal coronary angioplasty (PTCA) from January 1 through November 1 of the year prior to the measurement year, or who had a diagnosis of ischemic vascular disease (IVD) during the measurement year and the year prior to the measurement year and whose recent blood pressure is in control (< 140/90 mmHg).

NQF 0068
PQRI 204
Title: Ischemic Vascular Disease (IVD): Use of Aspirin or Another Antithrombotic
Description: Percentage of patients 18 years of age and older who were discharged alive for acute myocardial infarction (AMI), coronary artery bypass graft (CABG), or percutaneous transluminal coronary angioplasty (PTCA) from January 1 through November 1 of the year prior to the measurement year, or who had a diagnosis of ischemic vascular disease (IVD) during the measurement year and the year prior to the measurement year and who had documentation of use of aspirin or another antithrombotic during the measurement year.

NQF 0004
Title: Initiation and Engagement of Alcohol and Other Drug Dependence Treatment: (a) Initiation, (b) Engagement
Description: The percentage of adolescent and adult patients with a new episode of alcohol and other drug (AOD) dependence who initiate treatment through an inpatient AOD admission, outpatient visit, intensive outpatient encounter, or partial hospitalization within 14 days of the diagnosis and who initiated treatment and who had two or more additional services with an AOD diagnosis within 30 days of the initiation visit.

NQF 0012
Title: Prenatal Care: Screening for Human Immunodeficiency Virus (HIV)
Description: Percentage of patients, regardless of age, who gave birth during a 12-month period who were screened for HIV infection during the first or second prenatal care visit.

NQF 0014
Title: Prenatal Care: Anti-D Immune Globulin

Description: Percentage of D (Rh) negative, unsensitized patients, regardless of age, who gave birth during a 12-month period who received anti-D immune globulin at 26 to 30 weeks gestation.

NQF 0018
Title: Controlling High Blood Pressure
Description: The percentage of patients 18 to 85 years of age who had a diagnosis of hypertension and whose BP was adequately controlled during the measurement year

NQF 0032
Title: Cervical Cancer Screening
Description: Percentage of women 21 to 64 years of age, who received one or more Pap tests to screen for cervical cancer

NQF 0033
Title: Chlamydia Screening for Women
Description: Percentage of women 15 to 24 years of age who were identified as sexually active and who had at least one test for chlamydia during the measurement year.

NQF 0036
Title: Use of Appropriate Medications for Asthma
Description: Percentage of patients 5 to 50 years of age who were identified as having persistent asthma and were appropriately prescribed medication during the measurement year. Report three age stratifications (5-11 years, 12-50 years, and total).

NQF 0052
Title: Low Back Pain: Use of Imaging Studies
Description: Percentage of patients with a primary diagnosis of low back pain who did not have an imaging study (plain X-ray, MRI, CT scan) within 28 days of diagnosis.

NQF 0075
Title: Ischemic Vascular Disease (IVD): Complete Lipid Panel and LDL Control
Description: Percentage of patients 18 years of age and older who were discharged alive for acute myocardial infarction (AMI), coronary artery bypass graft (CABG), or percutaneous transluminal angioplasty (PTCA) from January 1 through November 1 of the year prior to the measurement year, or who had a diagnosis of ischemic vascular disease (IVD) during the measurement year and the year prior to the measurement year and who had a complete lipid profile performed during the measurement year and whose LDL-C < 100 mg/dL.

NQF 0575

Title: Diabetes: Hemoglobin A1c Control (< 8.0%)
Description: The percentage of patients 18 to 75 years of age with diabetes (type 1 or type 2) who had hemoglobin A1c < 8.0%.

Guideline #12

Patient Electronic Data Portal

Probably more so than any other guideline, this item is a large enhancement or change to existing workflows. This guideline requires that a facility provide patients with an electronic copy of their health information (including diagnostic test results, problem list, medication lists, medication allergies), on request. Ultimately this sets the course for the elimination of traditional paper-based records. Some systems implement this access as a web-based portal that can be used to access the information, others produce PDF files or other exportable documents that can be provided to a patient on a CD-ROM or other electronic sharing medium.

Measure

More than 50% of all patients of the eligible provider (eligible hospital's or CAH's inpatient or emergency department) who request an electronic copy of their health information are provided it within three business days.

Guideline #13

Comprehensive Visit Summaries

Provide clinical summaries for patients for each office visit.

Measure

Clinical summaries provided to patients for more than 50% of all office visits within three business days. The clinical summary needs to include a textual summary of the visit, coding and charge information, and as appropriate medications, labs, and other data.

Guideline #14

Clinical Information Exchange

The capability to exchange key clinical information (e.g., problem list, medication list, medication allergies, diagnostic test results) among providers of care and patient-authorized entities electronically. Many people in the healthcare industry, although David is not among them, see electronic clinical information exchange as a panacea of sorts, on one level to resolve problems of duplication in services and data, on another to provide a basis for analysis of data, and finally as a mechanism to improve patient care. Meaningful use strongly sets a foundation for future expansion of clinical information exchange by requiring support of structured data tracking and by requiring support for the CCD exchange format. In the current guidelines this one sets a very low bar for exchange, simply requiring support for the exchange format and that a single test be conducted. At the time of this writing it appears very likely that substantially more in-depth exchange will be necessary to be compliant in the coming years.

Measure

Performed at least one test of information exchange using the CCD (or related) format with another provider organization. For larger facilities this may involve use of a Health Interoperability Exchange (HIE) discussed elsewhere in this text. For most small and medium facilities completing the exchange can be done simply by utilizing some of the support required in other guidelines, specifically file encryption and CCD support. The facility can produce a CCD for a patient, encrypt it, and transfer it to another facility that also has a meaningful use compliant EHR system.

Guideline #15

Protect Health Information

Protect electronic health information created or maintained by the certified EHR technology. This is probably one of the least understood guidelines and in practice is not that large an undertaking for most organizations but on first appearance can seem daunting. The actual heart of this guideline is that as a facility you create a written policy regarding your passwords, access controls, and other electronic and physical measures you take to protect health information and then follow and conduct periodic audits of compliance to the written policy. The specific federal rules that must be reviewed go to pretty long lengths not to codify specific details of the policy that must be in place, only that there be a written policy and it is followed and audited.

Measure

Conduct or review a security risk analysis per 45 CFR 164.308 (a)(1) and implement security updates as necessary and correct identified security deficiencies as part of the risk management process. Implement standardized access, password, and logging policies. Conduct periodic audits against those policies to find noncompliance. The federal regulation is a bit difficult to digest but again the heart of it is just to take steps to create written versions of policies that protect health information and to follow those policies. It prescribes very little by way of what the policies your organization has must contain.

The preceding guidelines are all required. Each guideline and each measure must be compliant for a provider to be eligible to receive incentive dollars. In contrast, the following guidelines present a mix-and-match set that can be selected from. To be compliant, only 5 of the 10 guidelines and measures are required. At a minimum select the five most applicable to your line(s) of care, but there is much to be said for implementing compliance with more if you can. Each successive year will see more thorough and expansive guidelines, so it is better to get ahead of the curve if possible.

Guideline #16

Drug-Formulary Checks

Implement drug-formulary checks for at least one internal and one external formulary. There is often confusion about what exactly a formulary is. It is a preferential list of drugs, doses, and forms that can be put together by a facility to make prescribing more consistent. It is also published by payers to indicate drugs that are covered by their programs.

Measure

The eligible hospital's or CAH's inpatient or emergency department has enabled this functionality and has access to at least one internal or external drug formulary for the entire EHR reporting period.

Guideline #17

Lab Results

Incorporate electronic clinical lab test results into certified EHR technology as structured data. All major labs have various kinds of support for electronic importation of results. There can be problems if your facility works primarily with specialty labs or those that are regional or internal. To be compliant the results must be importable into the EHR's structured electronic data.

Measure

More than 40% of all clinical lab test results ordered by the eligible provider (eligible hospital's or CAH's inpatient or emergency department) during the EHR reporting period whose results are either in a positive/negative or numerical format are incorporated in certified EHR technology as structured data. Note that the relatively low threshold of 40% provides ample room for special cases involving regional or onsite labs that are not electronically importable.

Guideline #18

Patient List Reports

Generate lists of patients by specific conditions to use for quality improvement, reduction of disparities, research, or outreach. Of all of the pieces of meaningful use this capability and its potential strike us as the most underrated and most likely to have real-world benefits for patient outcomes. It is shocking just how little data analysis is done by facilities themselves and the capability offers a straightforward and powerful means to get facilities involved in looking at their own patient populations and important statistics about them. That introspection offers what might be the most promising avenue for significant improvements in patient outcomes with a minimum of effort.

Measure

Generate at least one report listing patients of the eligible hospital's or CAH's inpatient or emergency department, eligible hospital, or CAH with a specific condition.

Guideline #19

Reminders

Send reminders to patients respecting patient preference for preventive/follow-up care. Many facilities currently employ some process for reminding patients about upcoming interactions. This guideline brings into the electronic age the existing processes and is very synergistic with the patient lists of guideline requirements. This capability has the dramatic potential to improve patient outcomes with minimum effort.

Guideline

Measure

More than 20% of all unique patients 65 years or older or 5 years old or younger were sent an appropriate reminder during the EHR reporting period.

Guideline #20

Patient Access to Health Information

Provide patients with timely electronic access to their health information (including lab results, problem list, medication lists, medication allergies) within four business days of the information being available to the eligible hospital's or CAH's inpatient or emergency department. A supplement to the guideline regarding access to electronic visit information, this guideline expands that to the ability to provide a comprehensive record rather than just that of a current visit.

Measure

More than 10% of all unique patients seen by the eligible provider (eligible hospital's or CAH's inpatient or emergency department) are provided timely (available to the patient within four business days of being updated in the certified EHR technology) electronic access to their health information subject to the eligible hospital's or CAH's inpatient or emergency department's discretion to withhold certain information. For various reasons providers might choose to exclude certain classes or specific parts of records from this general sharing. Some states do have additional laws regarding access to legally complete records that might apply to this set of capabilities.

Guideline #21

Education

Use certified EHR technology to identify patient-specific education resources and provide those resources to the patient if appropriate. Facilities often have various mediums of patient education resources from videos to handouts and even websites. This guideline builds on the process by requiring documented and structured information about what education has been provided and what level of understanding the patient has regarding the resource.

Measure

More than 10% of all unique patients seen by the eligible provider (eligible hospital's or CAH's inpatient or emergency department) are provided patient-specific education resources.

Guideline #22

Medication Reconciliation

The eligible hospital's or CAH's inpatient or emergency department that receives a patient from another setting of care or provider of care or believes an encounter is relevant should perform medication reconciliation between the medication details provided by the other facility and any medication records at the currently treating facility. This process in most systems is done by recording the second set of medications as "outside reported" rather than prescribed or ordered and performing duplication, allergy, and contraindication checking among all those entries.

Measure

The eligible hospital's or CAH's inpatient or emergency department performs medication reconciliation for more than 50% of transitions of care in which the patient is transitioned into the care of the eligible provider (eligible hospital's or CAH's inpatient or emergency department).

Guideline #23

Summary of Care Record

The eligible hospital's or CAH's inpatient or emergency department who transitions their patient to another setting of care or provider of care or refers their patient to another provider of care should provide a summary of care record for each transition of care or referral. Similar to the other patient and electronic interchange guidelines, this item just ensures that information sharing is done in a compliant format when transferring patients to other care facilities or settings.

Measure

The eligible hospital's or CAH's inpatient or emergency department refers their patient to another setting of care or provider of care or referral care and provides a summary of care record for more than 50% of transitions of care and referrals.

Guideline #24

Immunization Registry Submission

Capability to submit electronic data to immunization registries or immunization information systems and actual submission in accordance with applicable law and practice. This guideline seems to have had the largest amount of errata and additional comment applied by CMS and other authoritative agencies. Although a valiant attempt to improve sharing of data with public health systems, implementation is severely hampered by the limited number and unique requirements of immunization registry systems present at most public health agencies. As a result the guidelines have been watered down to a point of reference only with the submission of very simplistic electronic data by existing means for a single test.

Measure

Perform at least one test of certified EHR technology's capacity to submit electronic data to immunization registries and follow-up submission if the test is successful (unless none of the immunization registries to which the eligible hospital's or CAH's inpatient or emergency department have the capacity to receive the information electronically).

Guideline #25

Syndromic Surveillance Data Submission

Capability to submit electronic syndromic surveillance data to public health agencies and actual submission in accordance with applicable law and practice. This guideline has suffered much the same fate as that regarding immunization registry submission with a number of comments and errata that erodes much of the potential benefit of this. A simple test can be conducted using a variety of formats that might or might not be of practical use. Only a single test must be conducted to comply.

Measure

Perform at least one test of certified EHR technology's capacity to provide electronic syndromic surveillance data to public health agencies and follow-up submission if the test is successful (unless none of the public health agencies to which an eligible hospital's or CAH's inpatient or emergency department submits such information have the capacity to receive the information electronically).

Inpatient Guidelines and Requirements

Although many of these guidelines are similar to those for outpatient facilities, there are enough subtle differences that they are listed here separately.

Because of the fluid nature of the meaningful use requirements and the ongoing rule making it is important to check with the registration website (*http://www.cms.gov/EHRIncentivePrograms/20_RegistrationandAttestation.asp*) for the latest information.

Guideline #1

Computerized Provider Order Entry (CPOE)

Use of CPOE for medication orders directly entered by any licensed healthcare professional who can enter orders into the medical record per state, local, and professional guidelines. This guideline covers ePrescribing as well as recording of medications that are dispensed and administered within the facility.

Measure

More than 30% of unique patients with at least one medication in their medication list seen by the eligible provider (eligible hospital's or CAH's inpatient or emergency department) have at least one medication order entered using CPOE.

Guideline #2

Drug Allergy Checking

Implement drug-drug and drug-allergy interaction checks. Typically this guideline involves both drug to drug allergy and drug to drug contraindications, although there is flexibility in the guidelines text in this regard.

Measure

The eligible hospital's or CAH's inpatient or emergency department has enabled this functionality for the entire EHR reporting period.

Guideline #3

Record Demographics

These include preferred language, gender, race, ethnicity, and date of birth. Some of those data points are tracked by most facilities but preferred language, race, and ethnicity are new demographics to many lines of care.

Measure

More than 50% of all unique patients seen by the eligible provider (eligible hospital's or CAH's inpatient or emergency department) have demographics recorded as structured data.

Guideline #4

Problem List

Maintain an up-to-date problem list of current and active diagnoses.

Measure

More than 80% of all unique patients seen by the eligible provider (eligible hospital's or CAH's inpatient or emergency department) have at least one entry or an indication that no problems are known for the patient recorded as structured data. Structured data here refers to the ability to report distinctly on individual problems by code. Clinical notes that might be recorded during a patient provider interaction are insufficient to comply with this guideline.

Guideline #5

Medication List

Maintain an active medication list detailing medications the patient is actively taking that are prescribed by the provider's facility or reported by the patient. Again this guideline requires data that can be reported on for each individual medication and cannot be complied with using only text clinical notes.

Measure

More than 80% of all unique patients seen by the eligible provider (eligible hospital's or CAH's inpatient or emergency department) have at least one entry (or an indication that the patient is not currently prescribed any medication) recorded as structured data.

Guideline #6

Allergy List

Maintain an active medication allergy list that tracks medication allergies at a minimum. All meaningful use certified systems to date also permit tracking of environmental, food, and other miscellaneous allergies as well as medications.

Measure

More than 80% of all unique patients seen by the eligible provider (eligible hospital's or CAH's inpatient or emergency department) have at least one entry (or an indication that the patient has no known medication allergies) recorded as structured data.

Guideline #7

Vital Signs

Record patient vitals as part of typical workflow including height, weight, and blood pressure; and calculate and display BMI and plot and display growth charts for children 2 to 20 years old, including BMI. This measure will be a significant workflow change for many types of facilities not accustomed to tracking vital statistics with this level of detail on each visit. A few select exemptions apply, so please check CMS advisories for more information. The reasoning for this measure even in lines of care where the necessity for vitals might not be immediately apparent is that vital statistics provide a solid evidentiary base for earlier prevention of the most problematic chronic diseases, and each interaction with a provider of any specialty is a good opportunity for this basic prevention step.

Measure

For more than 50% of all unique patients age 2 and over seen by the eligible provider (eligible hospital's or CAH's inpatient or emergency department) have height, weight and blood pressure recorded as structured data.

Guideline #8

Smoking Status

Record smoking status for patients 13 years old or older. Again this guideline applies to all specialties even if it has not historically been the case for this information to be tracked and even if it is not immediately obvious how it might be connected. Smoking-related illness remains a significant cause of adverse health and any interaction with a medical provider of any kind is a good opportunity to attempt to stop patients from smoking or to create correlating data about all types of illness and smoking.

Measure

More than 50% of all unique patients 13 years old or older seen by the eligible provider (eligible hospital's or CAH's inpatient or emergency department) have smoking status recorded.

Guideline #9

Clinical Decision Support (CDS)

Implement one clinical decision support rule relevant to specialty or high clinical priority along with the ability to track compliance with that rule. Clinical decision support remains the holy grail of EHR in many circles and is an advanced concept where the system can apply logical conditions to known data points and make recommendations or present evidentiary advisements about possible diagnosis, treatment, and outcomes for the patient. It is expected that CDS will play a larger and larger role as guidelines continue to expand in future years. This guideline provides enormous flexibility in how it can be complied with and sets a low bar with only the need to implement a single CDS rule, no matter how simplistic. To a large extent this guidelines is an indicator and placeholder to introduce facilities to the concept. CDS is a radical departure toward consistent and systematized care that is not that common today.

Measure

Implement one clinical decision support rule.

Guideline #10

Report Clinical Quality Measures

Report ambulatory clinical quality measures to CMS or the states. This guideline is the actual step of demonstrating meaningful use compliance by submitting the summarized numbers to provide compliance with each guideline.

Measure

For 2011, provide aggregate numerator, denominator, and exclusions through attestation to the state or federal government through the web-based reporting system. For inpatient facilities the measures are fairly complex and itemized here.

ED–1
NQF 0495
Title: Emergency Department Throughput—Admitted Patients. Median time from ED arrival to ED departure for admitted patients
Description: Median time from emergency department arrival to time of departure from the emergency room for patients admitted to the facility from the emergency department.

ED–2
NQF 0497
Title: Emergency Department Throughput—Admitted Patients. Admission decision time to ED departure time for admitted patients

Description: Median time from admit decision time to time of departure from the emergency department of emergency department patients admitted to inpatient status.

Stroke-2
NQF 0435
Title: Ischemic stroke—Discharge on anti-thrombotics
Description: Ischemic stroke patients prescribed antithrombotic therapy at hospital discharge.

Stroke-3
NQF 0436
Title: Ischemic stroke—Anticoagulation for A-fib/flutter
Description: Ischemic stroke patients with atrial fibrillation/flutter who are prescribed anticoagulation therapy at hospital discharge.

Stroke-4
NQF 0437
Title: Ischemic stroke—Thrombolytic therapy for patients arriving within 2 hours of symptom onset
Description: Acute ischemic stroke patients who arrive at this hospital within 2 hours of time last known well and for whom IV t-PA was initiated at this hospital within 3 hours of time last known well.

Stroke-5
NQF 0438
Title: Ischemic or hemorrhagic stroke—Antithrombotic therapy by day 2
Description: Ischemic stroke patients administered antithrombotic therapy by the end of hospital day 2.

Stroke-6
NQF 0439
Title: Ischemic stroke—Discharge on statins
Description: Ischemic stroke patients with LDL >100 mg/dL, or LDL not measured, or, who were on a lipid-lowering medication prior to hospital arrival are prescribed statin medication at hospital discharge.

Stroke-8
NQF 0440
Title: Ischemic or hemorrhagic stroke—Stroke education
Description: Ischemic or hemorrhagic stroke patients or their caregivers who were given educational materials during the hospital stay addressing all of the following: activation of emergency medical system, need for follow-up after discharge, medications prescribed at discharge, risk factors for stroke, and warning signs and symptoms of stroke.

Stroke-10

NQF 0441
Title: Ischemic or hemorrhagic stroke—Rehabilitation assessment
Description: Ischemic or hemorrhagic stroke patients who were assessed for rehabilitation services.

VTE–1
NQF 0371
Title: VTE prophylaxis within 24 hours of arrival
Description: This measure assesses the number of patients who received VTE prophylaxis or have documentation why no VTE prophylaxis was given the day of or the day after hospital admission or surgery end date for surgeries that start the day of or the day after hospital admission.

VTE–2
NQF 0372
Title: ICU VTE prophylaxis
Description: This measure assesses the number of patients who received VTE prophylaxis or have documentation why no VTE prophylaxis was given the day of or the day after the initial admission (or transfer) to the Intensive Care Unit (ICU) or surgery end date for surgeries that start the day of or the day after ICU admission (or transfer).

VTE–3
NQF 0373
Title: Anticoagulation overlap therapy
Description: This measure assesses the number of patients diagnosed with confirmed VTE who received an overlap of parenteral (intravenous [IV] or subcutaneous [subcu]) anticoagulation and warfarin therapy. For patients who received less than five days of overlap therapy, they must be discharged on both medications. Overlap therapy must be administered for at least five days with an international normalized ratio (INR) ≥ 2 prior to discontinuation of the parenteral anticoagulation therapy or the patient must be discharged on both medications.

VTE–4
NQF 0374
Title: Platelet monitoring on unfractionated heparin
Description: This measure assesses the number of patients diagnosed with confirmed VTE who received IV UFH therapy dosages and had their platelet counts monitored using defined parameters such as a nomogram or protocol.

VTE–5
NQF 0375
Title: VTE discharge instructions

Description: This measure assesses the number of patients diagnosed with confirmed VTE that are discharged to home, to home with home health, home hospice, or discharged/transferred to court/law enforcement on warfarin with written discharge instructions that address all four criteria: compliance issues, dietary advice, follow-up monitoring, and information about the potential for adverse drug reactions or interactions.

VTE–6
NQF 0376
Title: Incidence of potentially preventable VTE
Description: This measure assesses the number of patients diagnosed with confirmed VTE during hospitalization (not present on arrival) who did not receive VTE prophylaxis between hospital admission and the day before the VTE diagnostic testing order date.

Guideline #11

Patient Electronic Data Portal

Probably more so than any other guideline, this item is a large enhancement or change to existing workflows. This guideline requires that a facility provide patients with an electronic copy of their health information (including diagnostic test results, problem list, medication lists, and medication allergies), on request. Ultimately this sets the course for the elimination of traditional paper-based records. Some systems implement this access as a web-based portal that can be used to access the information, and others produce PDF files or other exportable documents that can be provided to a patient on a CD-ROM or other electronic sharing medium.

Measure

More than 50% of all patients of the eligible provider (eligible hospital's or CAH's inpatient or emergency department) who request an electronic copy of their health information are provided it within 3 business days.

Guideline #12

Comprehensive Visit Summaries

Provide clinical summaries for patients for each office visit.

Measure

Clinical summaries provided to patients for more than 50% of all office visits within 3 business days. The clinical summary needs to include a textual summary of the visit, coding and charge information, and, as appropriate, medications, labs, and other data.

Guideline #13

Clinical Information Exchange

The capability to exchange key clinical information (e.g., problem list, medication list, medication allergies, diagnostic test results) among providers of care and patient-authorized entities electronically. Many people in the healthcare industry, although David is not among them, see electronic clinical information exchange as a panacea of sorts, on one level to resolve problems of duplication in services and data, and on another to provide a basis for analysis of data and finally as a mechanism to improve patient care. Meaningful use sets a strong foundation for future expansion of clinical information exchange by requiring support of structured data tracking and by requiring support for the CCD exchange format. In the current guidelines this one sets a very low bar for exchange, simply requiring support for the exchange format and that a single test be conducted. At the time of this writing it appears very likely that substantially more in-depth exchange will be necessary to be compliant in the coming years.

Measure

Perform at least one test of information exchange using the CCD (or related) format with another provider organization. For larger facilities this may involve use of an HIE, discussed elsewhere in this text. For most small and medium facilities completing the exchange can be done simply by utilizing some of the support required in other guidelines, specifically file encryption and CCD support. The facility can produce a CCD for a patient, encrypt it, and transfer it to another facility that also has a meaningful use compliant EHR system.

Guideline #14

Protect Health Information

Protect electronic health information created or maintained by the certified EHR technology. This is probably one of the least understood guidelines and in practice is not that large an undertaking for most organizations, but on first appearance it can seem daunting. The actual heart of this guideline is that as a facility you create a written policy regarding your passwords, access controls, and other electronic and physical measures you take to protect health information and then follow and conduct periodic audits of compliance with the written policy. The specific federal rules that must be reviewed go to pretty long lengths not to codify specific details of the policy that must be in place, only that there be a written policy and it is followed and audited.

Measure

Conduct or review a security risk analysis per 45 CFR 164.308 (a)(1) and implement security updates as necessary and correct identified security deficiencies as part of its risk management process. Implement standardized access, password, and logging policies. Conduct periodic audits against those policies to find noncompliance. The federal regulation is a bit difficult to digest but again the heart of it is just to take steps to create written versions of policies that protect health information and to follow those policies. It prescribes very little by way of what the policies your organization has must contain.

The preceding guidelines are all required. Each guideline and each measure must be compliant for a provider to be eligible to receive incentive dollars. In contrast, the following guidelines present a mix-and-match set that can be selected from. To be compliant, only 5 of the 10 guidelines and measures are required. At a minimum select the five most applicable to your line(s) of care, but there is much to be said for implementing compliance with more if you can. Each successive year will see more thorough and expansive guidelines, so it is better to get ahead of the curve if possible.

Guideline #15

Drug-Formulary Checks

Implement drug-formulary checks for at least one internal and one external formulary. There is often confusion about what exactly a formulary is. It is a preferential list of drugs, doses, and forms that can be put together by a facility to make prescribing more consistent. It is also published by payers to indicate drug costs covered by their programs.

Measure

The eligible hospital's or CAH's inpatient or emergency department has enabled this functionality and has access to at least one internal or external drug formulary for the entire EHR reporting period.

Guideline #16

Lab Results

Incorporate electronic clinical lab test results into certified EHR technology as structured data. All major labs have various kinds of support for electronic importation of results. There can be problems if your facility works primarily with specialty labs or those that are regional or internal. To be compliant the results must be importable into the EHR's structured electronic data.

Measure

More than 40% of all clinical lab tests results ordered by the eligible provider (eligible hospital's or CAH's inpatient or emergency department) during the EHR reporting period whose results are either in a positive/negative or numerical format are incorporated in certified EHR technology as structured data. Note that the relatively low threshold of 40% provides ample room for special cases involving regional or onsite labs that are not electronically importable.

Guideline #17

Patient List Reports

Generate lists of patients by specific conditions to use for quality improvement, reduction of disparities, research, or outreach. Of all of the pieces of meaningful use this capability and its potential strike us as the most underrated and most likely to have real-world benefits for patient outcomes. It is shocking just how little data analysis is done by facilities themselves and the capability offers a straightforward and powerful means to get facilities involved in looking at their own patient populations and important statistics about them. That introspection offers what might be the most promising avenue for significant improvements in patient outcomes with a minimum of effort.

Measure

Generate at least one report listing patients of the eligible hospital's or CAH's inpatient or emergency department, eligible hospital or CAH with a specific condition

Guideline #18

Reminders

Send reminders to patients respecting patient preference for preventive/follow-up care. Many facilities currently employ some process for reminding patients about upcoming interactions. This guideline brings into the electronic age the existing processes and when combined with the patient lists guideline requirements is very synergistic. This capability has the dramatic potential to improve patient outcomes with minimum effort.

Measure

More than 20% of all unique patients 65 years or older or 5 years old or younger were sent an appropriate reminder during the EHR reporting period.

Guideline #19

Patient Access to Health Information

Provide patients with timely electronic access to their health information (including lab results, problem list, medication lists, and medication allergies) within four business days of the information being available to the eligible hospital's or CAH's inpatient or emergency department. A supplement to the guideline regarding access to electronic visit information, this guideline expands that to the ability to provide a comprehensive record rather than just that of a current visit.

Measure

More than 10% of all unique patients seen by the eligible provider (eligible hospital's or CAH's inpatient or emergency department) are provided timely (available to the patient within four business days of being updated in the certified EHR technology) electronic access to their health information subject to the eligible hospital's or CAH's inpatient or emergency department's discretion to withhold certain information. For various reasons providers might choose to exclude certain classes or specific parts of records from this general sharing. Some states do have additional laws regarding access to legally complete records that might apply to this set of capabilities.

Guideline #20

Education

Use certified EHR technology to identify patient-specific education resources and provide those resources to the patient if appropriate. Facilities often have various mediums of patient education resources from videos to handouts and even websites. This guideline builds on the process by requiring documented and structured information about what education has been provided and what level of understanding the patient has regarding the resource.

Measure

More than 10% of all unique patients seen by the eligible provider (eligible hospital's or CAH's inpatient or emergency department) are provided patient-specific education resources.

Guideline #21

Medication Reconciliation

The eligible hospital's or CAH's inpatient or emergency department who receives a patient from another setting of care or provider of care or believes an encounter is relevant should perform medication reconciliation between the medication details provided by the other facility and any medication records at the currently treating facility. This process in most systems is done by recording the second set of medications as "outside reported" rather than prescribed or ordered and performing duplication, allergy, and contraindication checking among all those entries.

Measure

The eligible hospital's or CAH's inpatient or emergency department performs medication reconciliation for more than 50% of transitions of care in which the patient is transitioned into the care of the eligible provider (eligible hospital's or CAH's inpatient or emergency department).

Guideline #22

Summary of Care Record

The eligible hospital's or CAH's inpatient or emergency department that transitions their patient to another setting of care or provider of care or refers their patient to another provider of care should provide a summary of care record for each transition of care or referral. Similar to the other patient and electronic interchange guidelines, this item just ensures that information sharing is done in a compliant format when transferring patients to other care facilities or settings.

Measure

The eligible hospital's or CAH's inpatient or emergency department refers their patient to another setting of care or provider of care or referral provides a summary of care record for more than 50% of transitions of care and referrals.

Guideline #23

Immunization Registry Submission

Capability to submit electronic data to immunization registries or immunization information systems and actual submission in accordance with applicable law and practice. This guideline seems to have had the largest amount of errata and additional comment applied by CMS and other authoritative agencies. Although a valiant attempt to improve sharing of data with public health systems, implementation is severely hampered by the limited number and unique requirements of immunization registry systems present at most public health agencies. As a result the guidelines have been watered down to a point of reference only with the submission of very simplistic electronic data by existing means for a single test.

Measure

Perform at least one test of certified EHR technology's capacity to submit electronic data to immunization registries and follow-up submission if the test is successful (unless none of the immunization registries to which the eligible hospital's or CAH's inpatient or emergency department have the capacity to receive the information electronically).

Guideline #24

Syndromic Surveillance Data Submission

Capability to submit electronic syndromic surveillance data to public health agencies and actual submission in accordance with applicable law and practice. This guideline has suffered much the same fate as that regarding immunization registry submission, with a number of comments and errata that erode much of the potential benefit of this. A simple test can be conducted using a variety of formats that might or might not be of practical use. Only a single test must be conducted to comply.

Measure

Perform at least one test of certified EHR technology's capacity to provide electronic syndromic surveillance data to public health agencies and follow-up submission if the test is successful (unless none of the public health agencies to which an eligible hospital's or CAH's inpatient or emergency department submits such information have the capacity to receive the information electronically).

Guideline #25

Advance Directive

Enable a user to electronically record whether a patient has an advance directive. An advance directive is a legal document often called an advance healthcare directive that is created by a patient or his or her legal guardian and instructs providers what actions they can and cannot take in the event the patient is no longer able to make decisions due to illness or incapacity, and appoints a person to make such decisions on his or her behalf.

Measure

Implement the capability to record whether a patient has an advance directive.

CHAPTER 9

A Selective History of EHR Technology

Health IT has a fundamentally different heritage from other IT systems. It will help you understand the products you're working with if you know the aspects of this separate linage, so we'll explore them here.

MUMPS: The Programming Language for Healthcare

The dawn of modern information systems is arguably the invention of the C programming language and Unix by Dennis Ritchie and others at Bell Labs. The C programming language and the Unix operating system gave birth to an industry that now includes Microsoft Windows, the Apple iPhone, and most of the other tech goodies that we know and love. Almost all software engineers are used to working on C-style programming languages. Even the physical layout of code (usually whitespace invariant) in modern programming languages is based on C.

Important attempts to computerize healthcare date back slightly earlier in the same era, which explains one of the central differences in health IT: MUMPS.

MUMPS stands for Massachusetts General Hospital Utility Multi-Programming System. It is typical nerd humor that a programming language sponsored by a hospital was named after a disease. Unlike C and Unix, there was no strong separation between the programming language of MUMPS and the operating system of MUMPS. In fact, originally, MUMPS was a programming language, database, and operating system all rolled into one. MUMPS was built by Dr. Octo Barnette in his animal lab and became the foundation of a hospital information system.

From the beginning, MUMPS was built to be a hierarchical database, rather than the table-based SQL databases that most programmers and information managers are familiar with. Until recently, this was something difficult to explain about MUMPS, but now databases with a similar hierarchical structure are on the market. Much of the recent NoSQL movement has been a return to design principles that have been in MUMPS for more than four decades.

As a fundamental data model, SQL works really well for data that is highly repetitive so that it can be well-modeled using a table. SQL starts to break down when the data structure varies greatly for each individual, which is the norm in healthcare.

MUMPS is significantly different from C-based languages. The syntax can be much terser, and it is not whitespace-invariant. This makes a block of MUMPS code look very intimidating to programmers who are not familiar with it—which is almost everyone. At one time there were several important vendors for MUMPS and the language was commonly used in finance as well as healthcare, but as the financial industry moved away from MUMPS the vendors consolidated. Now there are only two common MUMPS providers; Intersystems, which provides Cache, and the open source GT.M implementation. You might have seen Intersystems advertising an object database; they are talking about MUMPS. The name MUMPS was viewed by some commercial vendors as a marketing barrier, and as a result, they started calling the language M in an obvious reference to C. People who wanted to compromised between the original name and the market-friendly name often write [M]UMPS.

At least three of the most important health IT systems still available are based on the MUMPS programming language: MEDITECH, Epic, and VA VistA. VA VistA is the most widely feature-comprehensive EHR installed in the United States, running at every VA hospital in the country. MEDITECH, by many reports, is the largest proprietary hospital health IT vendor. Epic is generally regarded as the leading provider of health IT systems for very large hospitals. If you are running an EHR in a hospital in the United States, it is a good bet that you are running a MUMPS database.

Where Can We Buy Some Light Bulbs?

MUMPS is only one of the "shared histories" of health IT software vendors. One of the early revolutions in healthcare was the X-ray, which allowed people to see accurately the skeletons of people while they were still living.

As the value of X-rays to medical science became obvious, the technology was addressed by several companies with prior expertise in the required technologies—meaning that they made light bulbs. Later, the spread of computerization made it obvious that the photographic process in X-rays should be digitized, and medical imaging was the first area to be substantially computer based several decades before meaningful use began forcing normal doctors to computerize the contents of a medical chart.

The companies that had made the first light bulbs in the century before shepherded this early adoption of health IT and wrote software to run their various imaging machines. Usually, this software was the first enterprise software to run inside hospitals and clinics. It made sense for these same vendors to expand into general health IT. This is the reason why GE and Siemens are leaders in the modern health IT space.

Interestingly the companies that invested heavily in radiological systems also invested in early interoperability efforts around medical images. The resulting set of standards, called digital imaging and communications in medicine (DICOM), were among the earliest attempts to get different health IT systems inside hospitals to talk together. Originally, DICOM was used mostly to get different types of image sources (X-ray, MRI, CAT, etc.) to save medical image data to a central server. Eventually, it was understood that all of the different systems inside a large hospital needed to communicate, and the IHE efforts were born to define how each system should work together. IHE is a heavyweight, and comprehensive approach to healthcare information exchange. Generally, this means that the "light bulb companies" are often somewhat deeper into interoperability than other companies. For instance, General Electric employee Keith Boone, wryly dubbed motorcycle guy (*http://motorcycleguy.blogspot.com/*), is a full-time standards geek. He is often found either participating or leading efforts at IHE, HL7, Direct, and other standards bodies, and is one of the most outspoken advocates for good healthcare interoperability standards.

Fragmentation

For unclear reasons, no one health IT vendor has ever become dominant. A new company would start selling health IT systems, expand for a time, and then either stall out and shrivel up or become acquired by some other company.

The largest health IT vendor at the clinic level (and because 80% of healthcare happens in clinics, perhaps the largest health IT vendor of them all) is Allscripts. By some estimates, Allscripts has 15% of its market. But that 15% percent is not the result of organic growth. Today's Allscripts is the result of a merger between Misys and the original Allscripts, both of which in turn are the products of previous mergers.

All of this speaks to the most unusual aspect of the health IT market: its fragmentation. In other software industries, a clear winner usually emerges. For some reason, this has never happened in health IT. The large companies in health IT are either extremely old and grew very slowly, or they are the result of several mergers and acquisitions.

This process of acquisition has been accelerating in the face of meaningful use. Although the standards are fair, they do serve as an impediment to health IT startups and young companies. Many have chosen to sell their solutions to competitors, rather than bear the costs of certification.

In an Environment with Gag Clauses and No Consumer Reports

To establish a fair market, both the buyer and the seller must have access to the same amount of information. Economists sometimes call this concept *information parity*. In the market for EHRs, a typical vendor has substantially more information than any potential buyer.

This is particularly difficult to remedy. In other markets, Consumers Union provides the service of evaluating products fairly. *Consumer Reports*, which is published by the

Consumers Union, buys all of the products that it evaluates retail and does not accept payments from vendors in order to prevent bias in its ratings.

To do this with an EHR, an evaluating organization would need to have a hospital or clinic that it could use to install an EHR system and then uninstall it and repeat. Obviously, running a hospital merely to test EHR systems is not a viable approach.

There are several services that offer to provide insights into the performance of EHR systems. The most famous of these is KLAS (*http://www.klasresearch.com/*), which bills itself as "Accurate, Honest, and Impartial." Admittedly, they are honest in being open about receiving about 50% of their income directly from EHR vendors. But accepting money from the companies that they evaluate (which is the norm for the EHR evaluation companies) is not even the most significant issue with KLAS's evaluation method. The main problem is subtly tied in with their use of survey tools to have the technical leadership of hospitals and clinics evaluate the results of EHR deployments. That method tends to undervalue the impact of the EHR on front-line clinicians, and ignores important intangibles such as the financial stability of a given vendor. For instance, EHR vendor AcerMED was rated as "best in KLAS" by KLAS Research before being sued out of existence in 2007.

This is not to say that the KLAS organization does not live up to its moniker. In fact, they probably are accurate and honest, and to the degree that they are not impartial, at least they are transparent about their conflict of interests. The real problem is that the EHR industry is very difficult to evaluate objectively, no matter how honest the evaluator is. The danger with organizations like KLAS is that they give the impression of providing reliable data, when in fact their information might not actually help to establish information parity. It is reasonable to conclude that KLAS, and organizations like them, are doing the best they can. But their data is fundamentally limited.

One fundamental reason for the limitations on evaluators' data is the clauses in most agreements between proprietary EHR vendors and their customers, stipulating that the customer cannot discuss or criticize the product publicly, or even say how much they paid for it. In many ways, it's surprising that CIOs and other technical leadership at clinics and hospitals respond to the KLAS survey at all. Most contracts with EHR companies serve to ensure that the information parity needed to build a fair market can never reach the market. Indeed, only a small percentage of the information that KLAS gathers is ever publicly released.

There are movements within health IT seeking to overturn these types of gag orders, and it is possible that future versions of the meaningful use regulations will forbid these types of business practices. For now, it is very difficult to objectively evaluate the proprietary EHR marketplace, because most vendors want to keep it that way.

VistA History

In the late 1970s, a group of rogue programmers working at local VA hospitals began collaboratively developing software they called the Decentralized Hospital Computer Program (DHCP). Eventually, they were discovered by the central office at the VA and several of them were fired. This took the development process underground, ironically forcing the community of programmers working on DHCP to collaborate in a manner that would later appear in open source distributed development practices. People were free to use and modify each other's code, and the clinicians and programmers doing so spontaneously contributed their improvements back to the original author. This collaboration could not be centrally coordinated, because to do so might incur the wrath of the VA central office. This movement became known as the Underground Railroad at the VA.

Eventually, enlightened leadership at the VA discovered the work of the Underground Railroad and realized that this community had achieved what the central office had failed to provide for years: the skeleton of a system that could fully computerize healthcare delivery at the VA. The VA administration blessed the project and it was renamed VistA.

This group of rebel programmers not only eventually turned VistA into the most comprehensive EHR in the United States, but used it to drive forward the improvements that make the VA one of the most effective healthcare delivery systems in the world. This is the basic thesis of the book by Phillip Longman that we recommended in the introduction: *The Best Care Anywhere*. You can also read about the history of VistA (*http://www.hardhats.org/history/hardhats.html*) firsthand at HardHats.org or read a summary of the VistA project in the "What Is VistA Really" (*http://vistapedia.net/index .php?title=What_is_VistA_Really*) article on the WorldVistA sponsored VistApedia site.

Probably the most significant detail regarding VistA is that, because it was developed entirely by federal employees, it is available for download under the Freedom of Information Act (FOIA). Essentially that makes the source code for VistA available in the public domain. Public domain software can be used for the basis of both open source projects and proprietary projects.

CHAPTER 10

Ontologies

Practically speaking, an ontology is just a fancy word for a dictionary. More specifically, an ontology is a way of structuring knowledge, by coding complex concepts into simpler terms. Beyond that, ontologies vary widely in the level of complexity given to structuring the relationships between the terms. Some people use the term *ontology* in healthcare to refer to only systems that are capable of deeply modeling clinical information. Others use the term to refer generally to all types of abstract health care data sets. Sometimes, people speak about ontologies in terms of codes, code sets, or coding processes. This chapter will cover both important sources of clinical coding systems or ontologies, of several types.

The basic problem that clinical ontologies seek to address is the difficulty that automated processes have with synonyms. Heart attack, cardiac arrest, and myocardial infarction, as well as the acronyms MI or AMI, can all be used to describe the same event. Having multiple terms for the same thing is difficult if you want to fully automate any clinical information process. An ontology solves this problem by noting that the terms heart attack, myocardial infarction, MI, and AMI really are the same thing, and cardiac arrest, like cardiac arrhythmia are related terms, but not synonyms for those concepts.

Traditionally the academic study of ontologies has been of interest to philosophers, computer scientists, and cognitive scientists, who are deeply concerned with the mechanisms by which humans encode knowledge. We will mostly be ignoring the high-brow, but interesting, philosophical issues with ontology unless they specifically impact some aspect of the practical use of ontologies in healthcare. If you are already familiar with the concepts of ontologies you might be somewhat offended by the way typical medical ontologies ignore simple obvious principles that the science of ontology provides. Most medical ontologies are either irredeemably poor as knowledge representation schemes, or so consistently abused in practice that they might as well be. Moreover, no chapter on medical ontologies could begin without the admission that the coverage of ontologies is complex enough to merit a book on its own, and that the licensing of medical ontologies is so convoluted and inconsistent that this chapter certainly should not be taken as anything close to legal advice.

A Throw-Away Ontology

An easy way to get the basic concepts behind an ontology is to make up a silly, throw-away ontology, so that we can quickly understand the concepts involved. Of course, we will have to make up some utterly false health "facts" to go along with our discussion. We begin with the premise that foot size and type is critical to overall health. Once we accept this assertion, it becomes obvious that we need a way to clearly talk about foot size and type without ambiguity.

Almost all ontologies begin with elements in the form of a definition. Instead of only defining words, like dictionaries, we will define codes and phrases. For our example, we create series of codes to determine what big feet really look like, and our foot size ontology begins like this:

Big Feet
> Over size 15

Little Feet
> Under size 6

Normal Feet
> Between 6 and 15

Our ontology starts out informal, just a working consensus among us foot-health scientists. For this reason, we have limited ourselves to defining phrases. Now, at least informally, we all know we mean when someone says "Big Feet" in a foot-health diagnosis. But then someone points out that there is are clinical issues related to having a shoe size over 20, and that the European portion of our community uses a different standard, based on European foot sizes, that has somewhat different definitions of foot size, using European measurements. But the European foot-health ontology also defines the terms "Big Feet" and "Little Feet." How do we know when we are using the European ontology, versus the one that we are developing?

This problem is what computer scientists call a *namespace collision*, two things with different meanings, but the same name, occupying the roughly the same knowledge domain. If unchecked, this would lead to tremendous confusion, as one phrase might have two clinical meanings depending on who wrote it. This is a semantics error, and when people say "semantic interoperability" they mean transferable health data without this and other semantic errors. To fix this, we need to always specific which ontology we are using when we say "Big Feet."

We also recognize that we will need to make ongoing changes to the ontology as the science of foot health progresses. It is possible that we might need to redefine what the term "Big Feet" means when we discuss them today, versus what it means in the future.

To solve these problems we name our silly ontology and begin versioning it.

Fred's Fake Foot (FFF) ontology version 2.0

> *Really Big Feet*
>> Over size 20
>
> *Big Feet*
>> Over size 15
>
> *Little Feet*
>> Under size 6
>
> *Normal Feet*
>> Between 6 and 15

There is, of course, a competing ontology with the European alternative.

Silly Shoe Science (SSS) ontology version 1.0

> *Enormous Feet*
>> Size 40 and above
>
> *Big Feet*
>> Size 30 and above
>
> *Standard Feet*
>> Between 10 and 30
>
> *Little Feet*
>> Under 10
>
> *Hairy European Feet*
>> Hairy feet that Europeans often shave, causing blisters

As the fake foot science progresses, it becomes clear that there will need to be codes for the finger toe (that toe right beside your big toe). As it turns out, in our made-up world, having a finger toe longer than your big toe is clinically relevant. This makes some sense, because having a longer second toe is pretty freaky, even in the real world. So we extend our ontology to include two more "codes."

Freaky Second Toe
> A second toe that sticks out farther than the big toe

Normal Second Toe
> The second toe is smaller than the big toe

Next, we decide that we need to create codes and groups of codes so that we leverage computers to group patients with "strange feet."

Fred's Fake Foot (FFF) ontology version 3.0

> *9999 – Strange Feet Codes*
>> *9999A – Really Big Feet*
>>> Over size 20

9999B – *Freaky Second Toe*
A second toe that sticks out farther than the big toe.

1111 – Normal Feet Codes

1111A – Big Feet
Over size 15

1111B – Little Feet
Under size 6

1111C – Normal Feet
Between 6 and 15

1111X – Normal Second Toe
Second toe is smaller than the big one

Using the added codes and code families, we can quickly perform correlations between other health conditions and "strange feet." So far this ontology is a simple tree structure. More often than not, medical ontologies are too complex to encode as trees. As they mature they almost always turn into a web. In this ontology for instance, it becomes obvious that we need a more formal definition for "feet." We will call these codes "core" codes and so we will prepend them with a C.

C0001 – Foot:
The part of your body that touches the ground when you stand.

C0002 – Feet:
The plural of foot.

C0003 – Toe:
Things that stick out the end of a foot (C0002)

Now our ontology is a graph, illustrated in Figure 10-1.

Of course, because your authors have invested upwards of 10 minutes coming up with these ontologies, we want to protect the value of our labor and ensure that we have funds available to continue the important efforts of fake foot science. Therefore we publish the current versions of the ontologies with a license that ensures that individuals must pay a small fee to exercise the ontology copyright to communicate.

Learning from Our Example

At this point, we can now use our ridiculous ontology to begin discussing the real-world issues with ontologies.

First, ontologies are implicitly namespaces. The same terms can, and often do, have slightly different clinical meanings in different ontologies. Do not presume that two terms in English (or other languages either) are being used the same way in two different ontologies.

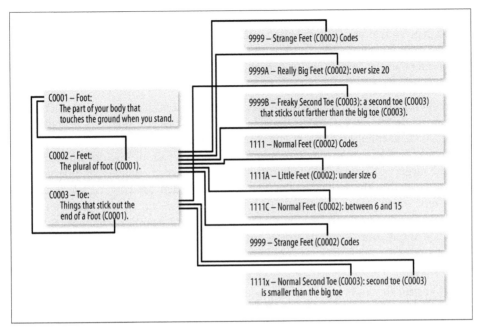

Figure 10-1. *HL7 standards*

When healthcare information encoded in one ontology needs to be used with health-care information encoded in another ontology, we have an ontology mapping. This mapping process is rarely perfect and should never be fully trusted. There are many ontologies, and efforts to create overarching maps between them are meta-ontologies. These meta-ontologies are necessarily clinically "lossy" because subtle distinctions between ontologies are often lost in large ontology mapping efforts.

We can also see, from our example, that health information coded with ontologies is often time-stamped. Foot size changes over time, so a person's foot code at age 6 is not likely to be his or her foot size later on.

Many of the useful ontologies have strict licensing agreements; they are owned by the organizations that develop them. Often, these organizations require payment for the use of the ontology. This creates a profit motive regarding the use of ontologies and as we have seen elsewhere in healthcare, strange incentives have strange results. If possible, proprietary ontologies should be avoided. Sadly, it is rarely possible to avoid them.

Versioning matters in ontologies. Data encoded with a code set in one year might have a different meaning when interpreted using the same ontology in a later version. Sometimes versions are backward compatible, but major revisions of ontologies should probably be considered a completely new ontology, in the sense that mapping is required in order to make the transition from one version of the codes to another.

Ontologies have sometimes significant geographic variations for legitimate reasons. Often different parts of the world have different encoding needs. Almost all internationally used ontologies have national subversions designed to address issues only found in given regions. Copyright and trademark law vary drastically between nations, and the rules for ontologies change with them. Most of this chapter will discuss things presuming that the context is U.S. copyright and patent law, which is usually the worst case scenario for practical health IT purposes.

Any ontology is based on some kind of scientific process. This example is, of course, entirely made up, but real medical science is often just as arbitrary. It is very difficult, for instance, to change the vocabulary of medical science for anatomy. Some body parts are named in Latin, many are based on the names of famous doctors who first conducted surgery on an area, and almost none of the scientific names for anatomy correspond exactly to natural language. The elbow and knee, for instance, are great summary terms for those joints, but those comfortable terms are rarely exact enough for clinical decision purposes. Remember just because your healthcare provider is talking with you about your "knee" pain does not mean that is how he or she is thinking about it. Your provider might discuss your "knee" pain but really be thinking "patellar tendonitis."

Good healthcare ontologies let clinicians make inferences on the clinical data sets encoded in them. For instance if we had 100 patients encoded with the FFF code 9999A Really Big Feet, we could infer that all of those patients also had 1111A Big Feet. This is a silly ontology that lets us make silly inferences, but useful and profound ontologies can help us make useful and profound inferences. The quality of inferences created by an ontology is the measure of the depth and clinical relevance of that ontology. Some people do not call a given data set an ontology unless it is capable of helping to make some kind of inferences.

Because medical language is fuzzy, and constantly changing, ontologies are fuzzy, too. Most ontologies are designed by committees of experts, and any information systems engineer will agree, design by committee rarely leads to the most effective designs. This fuzziness, and the fundamentally arbitrary process of assigning otherwise random numbers to clinical knowledge, leads us to one conclusion: ontologies are mostly arbitrary. The degree to which they are not arbitrary is the degree to which the ontology as a whole correctly models the state of medical science and the degree to which the ontology is leveraged in communication. It hardly matters if the model is better, without adoption. Like the metric versus English measurement systems in the United States, being better does not guarantee adoption.

Lastly, it is important to note that at any given point in time, even the best clinical ontology is going to be a snapshot of medical science at that given time. Medical science suffers both from mere wrongness and from societal bias. Countless procedures that are now known to be clinically useless or harmful could be easily encoded in the ontologies available when the procedure was popular. Bias in the healthcare community presents an even more troubling problem.

The *Diagnostic and Statistical Manual of Mental Disorders* (DSM) is the primary ontology of mental illness used in the United States. This mental health ontology was started by the American Psychiatric Association (APA) in 1952. In that edition of the DSM, homosexuality is listed as a mental illness. In 1957 Evelyn Hooker released the first extensive study that showed evidence that homosexuals were no less functional than heterosexuals. Over the next 15 years, more and more evidence would be released that homosexuality did not appear to impair the ability of a person to function in society. In 1973, under considerable protest, the APA removed homosexuality as a disease from the DSM ontology. It would take until 1986 to have it removed entirely.

Our example ontology is ridiculous, which in itself serves a purpose. A clinical ontology can be no better than the state of medical science that it reflects. Silly science in, silly ontology out. Remember that a clinical ontology is not the truth, just a reflection of scientific consensus. For the record, the second toe being longer than the big toe is called "Morton's toe" and it can actually have clinical relevance in some cases. Usually, it is just a normal variation and means nothing.

CPT Codes, Sermo, and CMS

Sermo is generally regarded as "Facebook for doctors." Although it is not clear that "Facebook for doctors" is even a useful idea, it is certainly true that Sermo is an extremely popular community and probably the largest doctor-only social network.

In May 2007, Sermo and the American Medical Association (AMA), the largest and most powerful medical association in the United States, announced that Sermo would become the official social media site for the AMA. As you can imagine, this was pretty big news (*http://www.sermo.com/news/pr/05/may/3/ama-and-sermo-enter-partnership -empower-physicians*).

In 2009 that relationship imploded (*http://www.kevinmd.com/blog/2009/07/the-ama -and-sermo-break-up-and-how-its-getting-ugly.html*).

A major part of the fallout was a blog post from the CEO of Sermo, Daniel Palestrant, regarding Current Procedural Terminology (CPT) codes. CPT stands for and is an ontology for medical procedures that the AMA developed. If you have read Chapter 3, you know that CPT procedure codes are the central ontology for doctors and hospitals to get paid in the United States.

The Sermo CEO wrote, in part:

> The current CPT coding system represents a collusion of convenience between the business side of the AMA and the insurance companies ... at the expense of physicians and patients. Perhaps most galling, thousands of physicians work on the CPT codes, for which they receive no compensation, while the AMA generates millions of dollars in revenue. Clearly this presents a massive conflict of interest as the AMA is supposed to be advocating for physicians, yet it receives the majority of its revenues from the very

same insurance companies that the rest of the physicians increasingly find themselves facing off against in the deepening healthcare debate.

Even more interesting than Dr. Palestrant's comment are the hundreds of Sermo posts from doctors commenting on the issue of CPT codes (*http://sermo.com/ui/blog/com ments/why_physicians_always_get_screwed.html*).

In 1983 the predecessor to CMS, the government agency that runs Medicare, dictated that providers who submitted bills to Medicare would need to code the procedures in CPT, and would need to code the diagnosis codes in ICD. This decision made CPT the de facto ontology standard for medical billing. Under the AMA's view, any healthcare provider can license the right to use CPT codes by purchasing that right from the AMA. You can visit the AMA website (*http://www.ama-assn.org/*) and purchase the right to use CPT codes for about $300 per year for one user. Obviously, bulk purchases can be cheaper. Under the AMA view, every provider who encodes information using CPT codes owes them money. As the Sermo CEO points out, the revenue that they get from licensing CPT codes outpaces income from membership dues, especially because membership in the AMA has been dwindling for years.

It might seem somewhat unfair that the government enforces the use of a proprietary billing ontology. Forcing all providers in the United States to use CPT codes is something like forcing all doctors to submit codes in Microsoft Word document format. Why should a private organization be the arbitrary beneficiary of a government policy decision without any opportunity for competition and alternatives?

You would not be the first person to feel that way. In 1997 in a landmark case, Practice Management Information Corp v. The American Medical Association, Practice Management Information (PMI) sought to show that because the federal government enforced the use of the CPT ontology, they should not be required to pay for the license to use the CPT copyrights. PMI lost the case. The judges ruled that because the government had chosen to give AMA a monopoly, rather than the AMA working to create one, there was no justification for invalidating the AMA copyrights.

It is not clear, to begin with, that ontologies can be the subject of copyright. Random numbering systems, at least, are not copyrightable. The famous court case Feist v. Rural regarding the copyrightablity of the numbers in a phone book established that copyright of mere facts, or mere associations between random numbers and simple terms, were not copyrightable. Before Feist v. Rural, a rule called "the sweat of brow" doctrine applied to U.S. copyright: if it took effort to generate a work, it was copyrightable.

Even before Feist v. Rural, mere information was not copyrightable. A mere fact, like "the sky is usually blue," cannot be subject to the protection of copyright. However, before Feist v. Rural, collections of facts were copyrightable. In Feist v. Rural, the court found that a phone book was essentially a collection of arbitrary facts, and therefore cannot be copyrighted. After Feist v. Rural, the new standard was creativity. Mere facts, or even collections of facts, cannot be copyrighted. Creative connections, ordering, and categorizing facts in useful ways can be copyrighted.

Medical procedures are simple facts. The way that the AMA encodes them is creative and therefore copyrightable. This is similar to the way a food recipe copyright works. A recipe is a set of instructions that is not copyrightable, but the words, sentences, and layout of recipes can be copyrighted. If you exactly copy a recipe from a cookbook and republish it, you might be violating copyright. But if you replicate the process described in a recipe in your own words, those words are not subject to the original author's copyright. Obviously just because the AMA owns an ontology for common medical procedures does not mean that they can lay claim to ownership of the procedures or alternative descriptions of them.

A procedure ontology is part mere fact (the procedures themselves) as well as creative work (the way in which the facts are encoded). This is an important distinction, because it deeply influences how ontology mapping can occur.

The other fact to highlight at this stage is that lawyers do not agree on what is or should be copyrightable. The old joke applies: Give two lawyers a legal question, and you will get at least three legal opinions. The copyright ability of ontologies is far from a closed question, as lawyers disagree about the issue and as knowledge science evolves, the courts will create further opinions. Perhaps most important, this discussion only applies strongly to an ontology that is primarily used in the United States. International health IT efforts are usually free to choose among inexpensive ontologies that require little or no licensing fees.

Returning to PMI v. AMA, the court ruled in favor of the AMA, in part because a medical ontology essentially has three components. The first component is a random code, which, by itself, is not copyrightable. The second is a short term like "Big Foot" that is close enough to a fact that it might not be copyrightable. The association between the short term and the numeric code, like the contents of a phone book, would not be enough to create a copyrightable work. However, if you include the longer text description of an ontology, then the combination of the three of them would probably be copyrightable. Moreover, the useful grouping of codes into blocks of relevantly connected codes is probably copyrightable. To review:

> 9999B – not copyrightable
> Freaky Second Toe – not copyrightable
> 9999B – Freaky Second Toe – probably not copyrightable
> 9999B – Freaky Second Toe: A second toe that sticks out farther than the big toe – copyrightable.
> 9999A, 9999B, 9999C, 9999D … 9999(x) all having to do with foot issues – copyrightable.

Should the AMA be able to own and license copyright to the CPT? Should CMS enforce the use of a proprietary ontology for medical billing? Is the Sermo CEO right that the AMA is protecting its CPT monopoly instead of advocating in the interests of the medical profession? Is this outline of the copyrightability of ontologies correct or is it missing subtle copyright issues? All of these questions are both fascinating and irrelevant to our current discussion of health IT.

What is relevant is that the AMA views the CPT ontology as an "intellectual property" (we use that term ironically) asset that it ferociously protects. A health IT vendor (PMI) went up against them in court and lost. As Dr. Palestrant notes, recent legislation supports and extends the CPT monopoly for claims transactions. Specifically, CMS is authorized under HIPAA to dictate what coding standards are used for medical billing. This regulatory power does not merely extend to claims submitted to Medicare. Bills to private insurance must also use the ontologies that CMS chooses. If healthcare providers want to use CPT codes in health IT software, and they must in order to legally bill third parties for healthcare services, they must license them from the AMA to avoid a legal fight.

Generally, health ontologies face difficulties with regard to licensing. Especially when more than one ontology is involved, the licensing implications can be very difficult to parse out. The Ontology Metadata Vocabulary (OMV) (*http://omv2.sourceforge.net/*) is an effort to make licensing and other "metadata" regarding ontologies clearer by providing a standardized ontology metadata format.

CPT licensing is not a trivial cost. A large hospital system might pay the AMA hundreds of thousands of dollars a year to license CPT codes. Small providers regularly ignore the AMAs licensing requirements (much like running pirated copies of software) and hope to slide under the radar of the AMA's enforcement. This can backfire drastically, and be an expensive mistake for a small practice. Unfortunately, this means that you, as the deployer of health IT systems, might be the first person to point out that the practice owes thousands of dollars a year in licensing fees to the AMA. Hopefully this section might provide you with the ammunition you need to convince a small healthcare practice to "go legit" regarding AMA licensing fees.

However, it is important to understand that although the AMA might believe that they have strong copyright protection over the CPT medical procedure ontology, they cannot have copyright to the mere facts of medical procedures. Moreover, the CPT terminology system is so focused on medical billing it is widely regarded as clinically impoverished.

The most significant impoverishment of CPT relates to its interaction with ICD codes. Before we further discuss the limitations of CPT codes for clinical purposes, we must discuss ICD codes.

International Classification of Diseases (ICD)

How do people die? In 1891, the International Statistics Institute wanted to formally answer that question and retire the numerous individual efforts that had pervaded this statistical inquiry for the preceding 200 years. Thus began (*http://www.who.int/classifi*

cations/icd/en/HistoryOfICD.pdf) the oldest formal medical ontology development process that is still in common use today.

ICD is a disease ontology. Disease here is used broadly to mean anything that has clinical implications that is the result of illness, injury, or is merely different about an individual. That is not the normal definition of disease, so most people refer to ICD codes as diagnosis codes, which is more accurate.

Today, the World Health Organization (WHO) maintains the ICD ontology. Older versions of the ontology are available in the public domain, and the current version can be used freely without costs.

The vanilla ICD database is not actually used in the United States, rather its cousin, the ICD-CM ontologies. The CM stands for "Clinical Modification," but it probably should be U.S. because the clinical modifications are actually intended to support disease concepts for U.S. medical billing. The ICD CM ontology is maintained by the Centers for Disease Control (CDC).

Claims data is composed of CPT procedure codes justified by ICD diagnosis codes. Together the combination of the two ontologies used in medical claims transactions forms a "billing ontology" that only applies to the United States.

E-patient-Dave-gate

As we mentioned in Chapter 6, the "e" in e-patient does not primarily mean "electronic patient," but "engaged patient" or "empowered patient." E-patients is a social movement that advocates for doctors and patients to abandon parental notions of healthcare. According to e-patients, all patients should take a more proactive role in their own healthcare and doctors and nurses should encourage this new empowered role.

One of the most vocal and famous members of the e-patient community is Dave de-Bronkart, who is better known as e-patient Dave. Dave used Internet research and collaboration with other patients to find a life-saving treatment for his metastasized kidney cancer. That amazing experience is not actually what made Dave famous.

In April 2009 Dave blogged about his experiences (*http://e-patients.net/archives/2009/04/imagine-if-someone-had-been-managing-your-data-and-then-you-looked.htmlO*) when he automatically imported his Beth Israel Deaconess records into Google Health, a personal health record. On April 13, 2009, the *Boston Globe* put Dave's story on the front page. Dave rocketed to international fame overnight.

Here is, in part, what Dave wrote about the contents of his Google Health record:

> The really fun stuff, though, is that some of the conditions transmitted are things I've never had: aortic aneurysm and mets to the brain or spine.
>
> So what the heck??

I've been discussing this with the docs in the back room here, and they quickly figured out what was going on before I confirmed it: the system transmitted insurance billing codes to Google Health, not doctors' diagnoses. And as those in the know are well aware, in our system today, insurance billing codes bear no resemblance to reality.

(I don't want to get into the whole thing right now, but basically if a doc needs to bill insurance for something and the list of billing codes doesn't happen to include exactly what your condition is, they cram it into something else so the stupid system will accept it.) (And, btw, everyone in the business is apparently accustomed to the system being stupid, so it's no surprise that nobody can tell whether things are making any sense: nobody counts on the data to be meaningful in the first place.)

E-patient Dave had stumbled on the first lesson of healthcare ontologies. CPT plus ICD claims data is mostly useless for clinical purposes.

This episode, which is nicknamed "e-patient Dave-gate" by health IT industry insiders, represented the first time that mainstream media recognized that claims data, given back to patients, creates lots of confusion. In the end, Beth Israel decided to stop sending any claims data to Google Health.

E-patient Dave was educated and intelligent enough to recognize that the "diagnosis" codes were not actually conditions that he had. Instead this occurred because of one of the dangerous interactions between ICD and CPT codes. Most of the reason for the "CM" part of the ICD code in the United States is that ICD is used to justify procedures. But many procedures are done as part of the diagnostic process. The simplest example is gall bladder removal. Often, patients have stomach pain that might be caused by the gall bladder, which can have disease states that are difficult to detect using modern scanning techniques. Each year many patients have their gall bladder removed without any evidence that the gall bladder is the source of the stomach pain. A surgeon never opens a patient up, looks at the gall bladder and says "it looks fine," and then sews the patient back up. If gall bladder surgery is initiated, the gall bladder is usually removed, even if it "looks fine."

The removal of a healthy gall bladder is often just a part of a diagnostic process. But when that procedure is billed to the insurance company, the diagnosis code that is given is probably ICD-CM 575.6, which stands for "unspecific disorder of the gall bladder." There is no code for "might be an unspecific disorder of the gall bladder." Many patients have the code 575.6 on their healthcare records that served to notify a health insurance provider of the reason for a gall bladder surgery, but in fact, the patient never had gall bladder disease at all, a fact that was only determined as the result of the surgery in question. The surgery must be paid for, hence the existence of the nebulous 575.6 ICD code, with a clinically unreliable meaning.

This is what had happened to e-patient Dave. He had gained access to his claims history, which is not the same thing as his healthcare record.

It is possible to use claims data to make determinations about clinical issues. Often, industry professionals can look at claims data for a single patient and infer what the healthcare record might look like. If they saw gall bladder removal, but then further treatment for stomach pain, they might infer correctly "gall bladder was never the problem." Further, data aggregation techniques can be used to mine large amounts of claims data for useful information. Insurance companies and government payers hire claims data analysis experts to mine terabytes of claims data for patterns. This process is a well-established health IT subindustry. It is surprisingly simple to detect and correctly infer clinically relevant information from such analysis, but no true health IT expert would ever presume deep clinical meaning in claims data alone.

CPT, combined with ICD-CM, was simply not meant for creating clinical records of care. Together, they form a "billing ontology" that is only relevant and useful in the contorted third-party payer system in the United States.

Generally, CPT codes are regarded as so billing-oriented as to be a clinically invalid procedure recording system. When it is used to justify CPT codes, ICD-CM is regarded with similar disdain. However, ICD alone, when used without intention to bill, could be a clinically valid diagnosis ontology.

When evaluating patient data coded in any ontology it is critical to understand both what the codes were made for and what they are used for.

Crosswalks and ICD Versions

The HIPAA mandated version of CPT is CPT-4. The current container version for electronic health claims is X12 4010A. The current version of ICD in the United States is ICD-9-CM.

Things change.

CMS makes determinations regarding which versions of both file formats and ontologies that healthcare claims in the United States use under HIPAA.

According to the current schedule, the container for electronic claims will change from X12 4010A to X12 5010 on January 1, 2012. More important, in October 2013, the current CMS schedule requires a change from ICD-9-CM to ICD-10-CM. Both of these changes will be extremely traumatic for the healthcare industry. Historically, CMS has frequently made last-minute extensions of deadlines like this, to accommodate the difficulty that many healthcare providers have shifting standards.

All translations like this create cottage industries of technologists who provide software or services to translate from the previously working standard to the current standard. Most health IT vendors will provide patches and mechanisms to enable their software systems to support coding in these standards, and many vendors already fully support both standards.

There are two major processes, besides simply supporting the underlying standards, that health IT professionals can look forward to.

The first is just the practical problems associated with teaching clinicians to use a diagnostic ontology that has close to 20,000 codes to one that has closer to 200,000 codes. Physicians have no training in medical school or in residency in the business of medicine, or science of coding (the kinds of things discussed in this chapter). For the most part, clinicians are using substantial mental shortcuts in the current billing process. Many times, a clinician checks a box on a paper form indicating what procedure was performed, and which diagnosis is justified, and very often, they check the same 20 or 30 options, day in and day out. Now, if that form is simply upgraded to cover the same code coverage, using ICD-10, that form would have to be the size of a poster. Obviously, that is not going to work and clinicians are going to need to learn to code diagnosis almost from scratch.

Until both the software and the clinicians understand ICD-10, there will be the continued generation of ICD-9 coded data. That ICD-9 data will need to be auto-converted into ICD-10 coded data in a partially automatic process. The basis of that process is something called a crosswalk or map. A crosswalk is a set of links between the same information in one ontology to another ontology. UMLS, which is discussed later, is essentially a merger of several crosswalks. For instance, both ICD and SNOMED CT are ontologies that can describe diagnoses accurately. It is possible to use an automated process, using a crosswalk as a map, to covert data coded in ICD to data coded in SNOMED. In this case, ICD-9 and ICD-10 might as well be totally different ontologies.

Thankfully, CMS makes this process much easier by providing very specific instructions regarding specific mappings in the form of general equivalence mapping (GEM) files available from the CMS ICD-10 website (*http://www.cms.gov/ICD10/*).

A substantial portion of the time, one ICD-9 code maps to one ICD-10 code. However, sometimes, one ICD-9 code could map to one of several ICD-10 codes (there is a reason there are more codes). In this case, determining which ICD-10 code is appropriate might require a quick review of a particular patient, or perhaps a working understanding of standard operating procedure for a particular facility.

Occasionally, several ICD-9 codes collapse primarily to one ICD-10 code. Most of the time, this occurs because a single concept has been completely remapped in ICD-10, and requires one core code, with additional codes to recapture meaning that is bundled in a single code in ICD-9.

The structure of the GEM files can be used to automatically detect which codes will need manual intervention.

Converting to ICD-10 will dramatically improve the capacity of CMS and other payers to understand what clinical conditions are being treated in particular patients. This will improve the richness and clinical reliability of claims data to a certain extent, which is good news for payers. However, patients and clinicians might not see much benefit from this change, especially immediately.

The transition from ICD-9 to ICD-10 will be painful as long as ICD-9 codes are being regularly converted to ICD-10 as normal part of the billing workflow. If possible, your organization should spend as little time as possible up-converting to ICD-10 codes or down-converting to ICD-9 codes. Unfortunately, the time when both ontologies will be used will be greatly extended by the fact that payers will also need to upgrade software to support ICD-10. It is possible that clinicians will have to create systems to support semiautomatic translation between the two ontologies for months or even years.

As a health IT specialist, you should become familiar with the resources and manuals associated with the CMS GEM files well in advance of your organization's migration requirements.

Other Claims Codes

CPT codes are entirely under the control of the AMA. CMS has been developing its own additional code set that is used alongside CPT codes to communicate other claim data. This code set is called the Healthcare Common Procedural Coding System (HCPCS). There are three levels of HCPCS, but the first level is actually identical to CPT-4. The second level is what are normally thought of as HCPCS, and the third level has been retired. For the most part, the levels of HCPCS serve only to confuse; when someone says HCPCS, they normally mean codes that are not included in CPT-4.

CMS, under power granted by HIPAA, mandates ICD and CPT/HCPCS for most medical claims transactions. It also mandates Code on Dental Procedures and Nomenclature (CDT) for dental procedures, and the National Drug Code (NDC) for drug descriptors.

CDT is largely equivalent to CPT codes, except instead of being owned, maintained, and licensed by the AMA, it is shepherded by the American Dental Association (*http://www.ada.org/3827.aspx*).

The NDC is maintained by the FDA and is a simple coded list of medications.

There are several other minor code sets that are required for very specialized medical claims transactions. These are documented on the CMS website (*http://www.cms.gov/educationmaterials/downloads/whateelectronictransactionsandcodesets-4.pdf*).

Drug Databases

NDC is probably the simplest drug database in existence. By itself, any mere list of drugs is pretty useless clinically. To be useful, a drug database should include as many of the following relationships between drugs as possible:

- Drug-drug interactions
- Drug-disease interactions

- Drug-food interactions
- Drug-treatment interactions

Of these, the drug-drug interactions are generally the largest interactions data set, and often people simple refer to the drug-drug interactions portion of a drug database to mean a drug interaction with anything. If it is possible that a drug could interact with anything in a patient's clinical environment, the drug database should include that information somewhere. For common interaction patterns, the drug database should enable automated querying to check against interactions.

Modern drug databases also frequently encode what pharmacists call ADMET, which stands for:

Absorption/Administration
How the medication gets in

Distribution
Where it ends up in the body

Metabolism
How it gets processed, and how fast

Excretion/Elimination
How it leaves

Toxicity
How much can kill or hurt people

The source data for drug databases worldwide is typically the U.S. government Department of Veterans Affairs' National Drug File (NDF). The VA hires many pharmacists to maintain a drug database. Those pharmacists add new drugs to the drug file, remove outdated and unavailable drugs, and maintain drug-ingredient interactions data. This data is merged with information on drugs that comes from the U.S. Pharmacopeia (*http://www.usp.org/*), which includes information regarding both drug and food ingredients, and lists from the FDA and the National Library of Medicine (NLM). All drugs approved for use in the United States engage in a back-and-forth process between the USP, FDA, and NLM, but the VA database contains drug data in a way that is designed to be used in a clinical environment.

Maintaining a drug database is thankless, difficult work that requires tremendous patience and attention to detail. Any given medication, illegal substance, or food will typically include several component substances. Not all drug-drug interactions are bad, and often new drugs are actually the combination of two previously separate drugs that are known to work well together. As a result, a drug database must concern itself with the fundamental ingredients of pills, injections, patches, sprays, and so on.

When any two drugs are prescribed together, a drug database must analyze all of the subcomponents of the drugs to determine if there is an interaction, and this process could potentially consider tens of combinations. When a patient has 15 or 20 medications, which is more common than you might think, drug interaction checking turns into a very complicated process. More advanced drug database integrations will also consider other components of a patient's health information, including conditions, treatments, and diet to ensure that other types of interactions are not occurring.

Not all interactions are created equal. Some interactions serve to make drugs more potent, and can sometimes be intentionally prescribed. Some interactions are weak, and in different clinical situations can be tolerated. Even major potential interactions might be acceptable in extreme circumstances.

Drug formats must be constantly updated. Often drug manufacturers will produce several doses of a drug, for instance, a 5 mg, 10 mg, 50 mg, and 200 mg pill. The next year, a manufacturer might retire the 50 mg pill and introduce a 20 mg pill.

The VA drug database is often biased toward the VA formulary. A formulary is a list of drugs that is available for purchase from a given health insurance provider or payer. The VA is typically its own payer, and as a result has its own list of which medications it typically offers. The VA, as a government agency, is focused on providing the information services that are valuable to the veterans in its care. However, as a government agency it is required to release software and data that it develops under the FOIA. Usually, for information that is requested by FOIA frequently, the VA simply posts the data on its website (*http://www.pbm.va.gov/NationalFormulary.aspx*) for download.

Several drug database providers download the drug database from the VA and maintain proprietary drug databases. To differing degrees, the drug database providers either use the VA data as a cross-check to their own independent drug research, or rely on the VA data as the core of their drug database product. The VA drug database is regarded as a correct but "messy" source of drug and drug interaction data. Most drug database providers ensure that the VA data is updated with information relevant to other formularies, and is otherwise clean and usable data, and then republish the data. Others use the VA database as a check against their own internal drug research process. Still others use the core ingredient data to make translations to other languages, where drugs are marketed under different names and potentially in different standard amounts.

The leading provider of proprietary drug data is First DataBank, which is owned by the Hearst Corporation. First DataBank sells a drug database to clinicians, usually through EHR vendors, and also engages in all kinds of drug-related data gathering and drug data analysis. It sells data to pharmacies, insurance companies, EHR vendors, and so on. It is deeply involved in the process for setting the prices for different drugs. There have been several lawsuits accusing First DataBank and the drug company McKesson of cooperating to artificially inflate the cost of drugs in the United States. Like much of healthcare in the United States, lack of transparent pricing for medications makes establishing a fair market very difficult.

Although First DataBank is by far the largest provider of drug data, there are several other drug database providers including Micromedex, MediSpan, Gold Standard Alchemy, and Multum. Each of these companies provides its own proprietary drug ontology, using a different coding scheme.

Thankfully, there is a meta-ontology that serves to map the different coding schemes of various drug database providers called RxNorm. RxNorm is maintained by the NLM at the National Institutes of Health (NIH). Well-designed EHR systems can support multiple drug database source data, and use RxNorm to reconcile differences between them.

RxNorm is the first component of the Unified Medical Language System (UMLS), which is a broad meta-ontology that unifies many different ontologies that we will discuss later.

Drug data, after claims data, is by far the most liquid data transferred in the United States. Most pharmacies in the United States are wired to accept prescriptions electronically. This is largely the result of the Surescripts network. Surescripts is the result of a 2008 merger of the only two large e-prescribing providers in the United States, RxHub and the original, smaller Surescripts. As a result of this merger, Surescripts has near-monopoly status on the routing of electronic prescriptions in the United States. Meaningful use requires e-prescribing. Technically, this does not mandate integration with Surescripts, but practically Surescripts is required. Surescripts is the only way to ensure that electronic prescriptions actually reach pharmacies. Eventually, the Nationwide Health Information Network (NWHIN) will provide an alternate pathway between clinicians and pharmacies. As pharmacies realize that the use of the new network would essentially be free, compared with Surescripts, which charges substantial fees, NWHIN adoption for e-prescribing could quickly become very popular. With companies like NewCrop (described later) in a position to make a profit advantage of such a second e-prescribing pathway, the competitive landscape could shift substantially in coming years.

Electronic prescribing requires the merger of at least three different healthcare ontologies and databases. The first is a drug database, keyed to RxNorm. The second and third are healthcare provider identification schemes, the National Provider Identifier (NPI) mandated by HIPAA for medical claims transactions, and Drug Enforcement Agency (DEA) number that is given to doctors, dentists, veterinarians, and anyone else with the privilege to prescribe controlled substances. Historically there has been considerably paranoia regarding the electronic prescription of controlled substances. The DEA and HHS together maintain the controlled substances list, and knowing the shorthand for controlled substances is important for electronic prescribing:

- Schedule 1: Drugs with no medical use that are very addictive, like heroin.
- Schedule 2: Drugs with limited medical use that are very addictive, like morphine.
- Schedule 3: Drugs with a little more medical use, and a little less addictive than Schedule 2, like steroids.

- Schedule 4: Drugs with a little more medical use, and a little less addictive than Schedule 3, like phenobarbitol.
- Schedule 5: Drugs with a little more medical use, and a little less addictive than Schedule 4, like codeine in cough suppressant.

The drug schedule does not make sense, and likely never will. For instance, the street drug heroin is Schedule 1, which makes sense, but cocaine, another dangerous street drug, is Schedule 2. Marijuana is Schedule 1, but is currently quasi-legal to prescribe by state law in California and some other states. The important lesson here: all drugs are somewhere on the schedule (except alcohol and tobacco, which are regulated separately by the ATF), the schedule determines how prescriptions can be written, and you should never, ever guess what schedule a medication is. This is information that you should get from your drug database.

Until recently, prescribing "serious" low-schedule medications could not be done using electronic prescribing. This rule, which has stunted the uptake of e-prescribing by forcing doctors to have both a paper prescribing and e-prescribing process in parallel, has now been relaxed assuming certain digital signatures are in place. Practically speaking, these digital signatures and the biometrics processes that are typically involved with them will become a requirement, either through meaningful use, or through practical necessity.

The most significant rule regarding drug databases is that they should never be trusted for tasks that they are not doing, and they should constantly be updated. New drug interactions, even involving older drugs, are discovered all the time. Using an outdated drug interaction file can expose your organization to serious liability. Further, if you purchase a drug database that has drug-drug interactions, but does not include drug-food interactions, then it is critical that clinical staff understand that the health information system is incapable of catching food-drug interactions.

There are several other drug-related databases that are worth mentioning: The WHO maintains an ontology of adverse drug reactions (*http://www.who.int/medicines/areas/quality_safety/en/*) that describes what can go wrong with different medications.

Dailymed (*http://dailymed.nlm.nih.gov/*) is a database of the contents of medication inserts (the several pages of really small text that you never read on the inside of your prescriptions) that comprehensively describes a given medication.

HL7 publishes a standard for labeling products called Structured Product Labeling (SPL) (*http://labels.fda.gov/*) that the FDA uses to publish the labels for drugs.

Electronic prescribing is a powerful tool, but it is often underutilized. The Surescripts network is capable of feeding your EHR data regarding what medications a patient has been prescribed elsewhere. It is critical that this data be properly imported into your EHR to properly check for drug interactions. This should occur at the pharmacy also, but often does not.

In many cases, however, e-prescribing will represent new burdens on doctors. E-prescribing requires very specific details regarding dose, dose form, drug form, and countless other details. These details are defined by the National Council for Prescription Drug Programs (NCPCP). With e-prescribing, for instance, a clinician will have to specify whether a drug should be a capsule or a tablet, and whether generic equivalents are acceptable. With paper prescriptions many of these details were determined by the pharmacists and patients. E-prescribing is an entirely new skill set.

One of the important players in the e-prescribing space is a low-profile company called NewCrop. NewCrop provides an integration layer to e-prescribing and automatically faxes prescriptions that cannot be delivered using the Surescripts network. NewCrop provides at least two different integration methods for EHR systems. The first is an API for deep integration. This allows an EHR to appear to be doing e-prescribing, but allows NewCrop to do the heavy lifting. The other, simpler integration allows web-based EHR systems to hand off users to a NewCrop web interface, so that NewCrop actually provides the user interface to e-prescribing. NewCrop is essentially a drug ontology merging shop, providing unified drug ontology licensing services as well as substantial services mapping plain text drug data (from a doctor's typed note for instance), onto proper drug ontologies. Given the number of standards and protocols involved in e-prescribing, this is regarded as a very valuable service. Most small EHR vendors use NewCrop to ease the complex integration with Surescripts. When searching the Surescripts website (*http://www.surescripts.com/connect-to-surescripts/prescriber-software/search .aspx*) for certified vendors, NewCrop clients show up with "Uses NewCrop" under their product name.

MirrorMed, an open source EHR feeder project for ClearHealth, contains a reference open source implementation of the NewCrop interface (*http://mirrormed.svn.source forge.net/viewvc/mirrormed/modules/newcrop/*) as an add-on module to ClearHealth.

SNOMED to the Rescue

If there was a "winner" in the clinical ontology space it would be SNOMED CT, which stands for Systematized Nomenclature of Medicine – Clinical Terms.

If there was a clinical specialty that could be regarded as responsible for "classifying" medicine, it would be pathologists. Pathologists are doctors who specialize in running laboratory tests on human tissue and fluids. Pathologists can often spend much of their career looking through a microscope or using other lab equipment. Because they often provide diagnoses that are unreachable in any other way, pathologists have the nickname of "the doctor's doctors."

In the United States, one of the respected professional organizations for pathologists is the College of American Pathologists (CAP). Since the late 1960s, CAP had been working on a clinically accurate ontology that could be broadly applied to all aspects of medicine. In 1997, the trademarks and copyright for SNOMED were transferred to a new international body called the International Health Terminology Standards Development Organization (IHTSDO). In 1999 SNOMED was merged with similar efforts from the United Kingdom Clinical Terms project. The result is SNOMED CT, which is generally regarded as the most complete clinical ontology in any language.

Moreover, SNOMED CT is liberally licensed to any IHTSDO "member country." Because the main ontology was created in English, this list includes the United States, Canada, the United Kingdom, and Australia. Several other European countries participate in IHTSDO, but adoption is far from universal, focusing on North American and European countries. Recently, IHTSDO has decided to liberally license SNOMED CT to very poor countries free of charge. If a nation is defined as poor by the World Bank, they can use SNOMED CT as if they were a member country. International readers, especially in non-English-speaking middle-income or wealthy countries should verify the status of their nation in the IHTSDO member list (*http://ihtsdo.org*). If you are not in an IHTSDO member country or in a country treated as a member country you might need to pay licensing fees to use SNOMED CT.

Because so many people have free access to SNOMED CT, it has rapidly become the de facto standard for encoding health information in a clinically valid way, and is regarded as the "right" way to populate popular health information exchange formats such as CCR/CCD/CDA (acronyms explained in Chapter 11).

SNOMED Example

Because SNOMED is so popular, an example of the coding scheme is warranted. Suppose a patient dropped boiling water on his or her left foot that resulted in second-degree burns. In SNOMED, that could be encoded as:

Concept ID = 62537000
Fully Specified Name = Second-degree burn of foot

This code has certain relationships with other codes, like its parents, which include:

37696000 Burn of lower leg
125604000 Injury of foot

In turn, this code has a parent code:

84677008 Burn of the lower limb

It has an "associated morphology" of

46541008 Second-degree burn injury

and a "finding site" of

60496002 Skin structure of the foot

For any given instance of a foot burn, you might also have codes that further specify when it happened, how often it happens, what type of person provided the information, and so on.

Most important, it should be noted that if the core concept for "Second-degree burn of the foot" were missing from SNOMED, it could be largely re-created by grouping other codes together. This allows SNOMED to describe things accurately that it does not directly encode.

SNOMED uses a complex method of coding. Each number (formally called a SNOMED CT identifier or SCTID) has a structure that can be used by a computer system to make determinations about which particular part of SNOMED the SCTID comes from. It also includes a check digit to protect against data entry mistakes. A computer can use an algorithm to determine if an SCTID that was typed in is valid. For the most part, typing SCTIDs should be avoided in any case. From a user's standpoint, they should almost always be seeing the descriptions instead. Similarly, searching via SCTIDs is only something done during data analysis, so casual searches will almost always focus on the descriptions. SCTIDs are random numbers at this stage, and do not reflect the structure of SNOMED CT, although this might change someday.

Relationships are also rarely used extensively by front-end users (at least not overtly). Instead when relationships are good for doing analysis on patient records, and driving intuitive user interfaces for clinical users. So your end users will never directly care that a "surgery" is a "procedure," or that 37696000 is a parent of 62537000, but you as a data engineer certainly might. These relationships allow SNOMED CT to not merely code medical knowledge, but participate in the development of new clinical information via inferences.

Dr. Hendler regularly provides the following example in presentations:

> Pneumococcus "Is A" type of Gram Positive Coccus. Gram Positive Cocci "Is A" type of bacteria. Streptococcus "Is A" different kind of Gram Positive Coccus.
>
> Strep throat "Is A" disease. It has findingSite pharynx, it has morphology inflammation, and it has causativeAgent Streptococcus.
>
> Pneumococcal Pneumonia "Is A" different disease. It has findingSite Lung Structure, it has morphology inflammation and it has causativeAgent Streptococcus.
>
> For the sake of argument (this is made up), let's say that you come to suspect that anyone with any Gram Positive Coccal infection who was treated with a certain class of antibiotic later develops kidney disease. You would need to find all the patients who had Gram Positive Coccal infections. Using lexical searching or ICD9 you could not do this in a systematic way. You would just have to know every possible name for a condition, and every possible organ system that might be involved.
>
> You would certainly miss some relevant conditions. SNOMED CT allows you to do a "subsumption" search. You can ask the reasoner (software that queries ontologies) to find for all SNOMED CT codes in the set:
>
> All diseases with causative agent Gram Positive Cocci.

It will not only find the two conditions listed above but many more, some of which a typical physician has probably never heard of. Then, after the reasoner returns a comprehensive list of codes that match your search criteria, you can take that list and use it to query your EHR. This provides a list of patients who have symptoms or diseases that could be caused by Gram Positive Cocci. You further restrict that list to see who has received the antibiotic in question, and now you have a data set which addresses your hypothesis regarding kidney disease.

This example demonstrates how an ontology such as SNOMED CT, which encodes a much deeper level of medical knowledge than billing ontologies, can provide clinicians with information and context that is simply impossible without a robust ontology.

SNOMED CT has more than 300,000 terms in its ontology. It has millions of relationships between those terms. In comparison, ICD-10 numbers about 150,000 concepts, up from around 17,000. Practically speaking this means that you cannot "buy the SNOMED book" in the way that you can with ICD and CPT codes. We will discuss in the next section some of the implications of dealing with an ontology of that size from a technical standpoint.

From a practical standpoint, SNOMED's size is both one of its greatest strengths, as it is by far the most comprehensive clinical ontology available, but also its weaknesses, as mistakes in the ontology are difficult to find and fix.

SNOMED CT can be downloaded with UMLS from the NLM (*http://www.nlm.nih.gov/ research/umls/*).

SNOMED and the Semantic Web

This section contains a technical discussion of how queries work on data encoded using SNOMED. If that subject does not interest you, we recommend you skip this section and come back to it when you need it.

Computers are very very good at repetitive processes. Modern desktop computers can perform millions of simple calculations in the time it takes to blink. Those simple calculations can add up to more complex calculations, which gives us the broad range of things that computers can do. Still, we all have experienced our computers slowing down when performing complex tasks, especially on large data sets.

The science of how hard it is for a computer to calculate something, based on the size of the data set required, is called *computational complexity*. Computational complexity is far beyond the scope of this book, except to outline the basics of the concept. Basically computational complexity varies greatly depending on the size of the data set in question. If a computational process is very efficient, then there is little increase in the amount of computing required when a data set gets larger.

This is like the famous chessboard and wheat problem. If you place a single grain of wheat on the first square, and then double that, and place 2 on the next, and continue with 4, 8, 16, 32, 64, and so on, you end up with 18,446,744,073,709,551,615 grains of wheat in total, or a pile of wheat the size of Mount Everest. If you view each additional square as a new data point, and the grains of wheat as the computational cycles required to process that data point, you begin to see the potential problem with computational complexity.

SNOMED is a very large ontology. When a large clinical data set, say 10,000 patient records, is encoded using SNOMED, the computational task to query those patient records based on SNOMED relationships might easily have become a wheat-grain task.

However, SNOMED CT is conformant to OWL 2 EL. OWL stands for Web Ontology Language and is the standard of choice for semantic web. OWL 2 EL is subset of the OWL language that intentionally restricts some semantic relationships (negation and disjunction specifically) that make querying extremely large data sets something that computers can do more easily.

SNOMED CT has had growing pains over the years in terms of its "semantic goodness," but its compliance with OWL 2 EL means that many of the modern tools that apply to OWL can be leveraged to perform data analysis on SNOMED encoded clinical data. Moreover, full, usable OWL compliance might not be too far off, given advancing processing speeds and improved OWL tools along with improvements to the SNOMED ontology. A new OWL reasoner, called the *condor reasoner (http://code.google.com/p/ condor-reasoner/)*, has been especially productive in processing SNOMED CT. We can recommend the book *Programming the Semantic Web (http://oreilly.com/catalog/ 9780596153816)*, by Toby Segaran, Colin Evans, and Jamie Taylor (O'Reilly), to help you determine what you can make of SNOMED's OWL compliance.

To actually get SNOMED files into OWL formats, you can use a Python script from the clinical ontology modules of the python-dlp (*http://code.google.com/p/python-dlp/ source/browse/trunk/clinical-ontology-modules?spec=svn319%38r=319*) project, or Perl scripts written by Kent Spackman, included in the UMLS distribution of SNOMED CT under the "Other Resources/Developer Toolkit" directory. Both of these tools will provide an OWL output of SNOMED that can be used for the basis of other queries. You might also consider using some of the ontology management tools mentioned later in the chapter.

UMLS: The Universal Mapping Metaontology

This chapter has provided a tour of important ontologies in medicine. We have considered several drug ontologies, which are mapped together using RxNorm. We have considered CPT and ICD codes, which form the heart of a patient's claim history. And we have considered SNOMED, which is a comprehensive and available clinical ontology.

But we know that there is considerable overlap in all of these ontologies. There is also overlap between different versions of these ontologies, as we see in the transition between ICD-9 and ICD-10.

There is a project whose sole existence is to map the meanings between different clinical ontologies worldwide. That ontology, which is really a meta-ontology, is called the UMLS. If Frodo were carrying an ontology, it would be UMLS. It is absolutely the one ring to bind them. The heart of UMLS is its metathesaurus. The metathesaurus is the end result of the use of other UMLS components, which largely exists to create this metathesaurus.

The metathesaurus includes semantic concepts that are mapped onto other ontology systems. There are 2 million concepts in UMLS, but they map onto around 200 ontologies. Many of these ontologies are in languages other than English and some are in several languages. Although almost 70% of the descriptions are in English, the translation of medical terminology is an important concept embedded in UMLS.

Many of the ontologies that are "wrapped up" in UMLS contribute only a few hundred or thousand concepts. But massive ontologies like SNOMED, ICD, and CPT ensure that there are many many concepts in the UMLS database. RxNorm, for instance, is merely the drug database component of the larger UMLS meta-ontology.

The licensing for UMLS can be very complicated, because it involves sublicensing the various subcomponents. It is possible only to use a subset of UMLS that includes ontologies that you want to license. However, in some cases, licensing an expensive ontology through UMLS can have unexpected financial benefits.

Many organizations use the capacity of UMLS to map SNOMED to CPT codes to avoid paying expensive licensing fees to the AMA. A large organization will have its clinicians code procedures using SNOMED CT, which costs nothing for providers to use in the United States. Hundreds of clinical users can code in SNOMED without needing to pay any fees to the AMA. Then, using UMLS, medical billing specialists translate the procedures into CPT codes just for billing. Assuming only a few billing specialists perform this task, the licensing codes for CPT are minimal at best.

It is important that any organization considering this strategy do so carefully. All medical claims must be fully justified by the contents of the clinical record, and using the shift between SNOMED to CPT to illegally upcode can be an expensive mistake. Alternatively, downcoding for safety can also result in lost income.

More than just a potentially direct financial benefit, UMLS holds the key to true semantic interoperability. It is only when the underlying meaning in each ontology can be mapped to the meaning in another ontology, even in another language, that we can hope for worldwide semantic interoperability of healthcare records.

Extending Ontologies

As a rule, ontologies all have an associated standards body, through whom additions and extensions to a given ontology are managed. Often, a clinical organization that is using an ontology to drive clinical workflows will feel the need to add a code to an ontology. This should generally be avoided because adding codes with meanings that only your clinic or hospital understands makes fully semantic interoperability much more difficult. No other organization will be able to parse clinical data encoded in this way.

There are two general reasons this happens.

First, it is possible, especially in research-oriented clinical environments, to find that a new code is clinically justified. That is to say, existing codes or combinations of codes in a given ontology might fail to capture some significant clinical meaning that should be captured in a formal way, in relation to the ontology. This is a legitimate reason to add a code, but most ontologies have a process by which an organization can create a temporary code and have that code submitted to become part of the larger ontology through some kind of approval process. This case surfaces a legitimate reason to extend ontologies, but follow-through is important.

Care should be taken to ensure, when an ontology is extended for clinical purposes, formal coordination with the standards body that manages the given ontology. In many cases, your request for additional codes will be denied, but rarely will this happen without the standards body taking your clinical use case into consideration and addressing it in some other way. If the standards body does ultimately deny your request for a new code, and provide an alternative means of coding your clinical use case, the codings using the old code should be updated to include the new coding schema. This is the only way to ensure that new clinical meaning generated at your specific site does not ultimately contribute to the breakdown of semantic interoperability.

The other reason people extend medical ontologies happens when part of the workflow requires a trigger that is different than the triggers already provided by the available codes. It is common for an automated workflow to have rules like "Whenever a patient coded with this CPT code goes to an X-ray, do ABC." However, a well-designed EHR should have mechanisms in place to support workflow modification without adding workflow-related codes into your local copy of an ontology. It is critical that the purpose of the ontology be focused on coding clinical data. Even billing ontologies, like CPT, should never be extended with data that is clinically meaningless outside your organization. A good rule of thumb is that an additional, custom code is acceptable for clinical reasons but not for workflow reasons.

Many practice management systems, or EHR systems that grew from practice management systems, rely on additional custom codes in the CPT database to function. This is a dangerous design flaw, and software that does this should be avoided or repaired if possible.

Other Ontologies

The fourth edition of the *Diagnostic and Statistical Manual of Mental Disorders* (DSM IV) is the current way for mental health providers to code behavioral disease. The DSM

V will be released in 2013. As we mentioned in the introduction, the DSM is often a controversial place where hot-button cultural issues play out. Mental health disease still has considerable stigma associated with it in the United States, and the DSM is often the battleground where arguments regarding perception take place.

Furthermore, mental health is one of the few endeavors where the name of your formal diagnosis might actually have impacts on your real-world health. Hearing that you have "mild" depression, rather than "major" depression, for instance, might actually impact how depressed you feel. All of this makes DSM one of the most important and high-impact healthcare ontologies available.

Mental health issues are often coded in other, general-purpose ontologies like ICD and SNOMED, making UMLS especially important for mental health coding purposes.

Cyc is a an artificial intelligence project that is attempting to build a very comprehensive ontology for everything, and not just for healthcare. OpenCyc is an open source release of Cyc that has some reduced capacity. Although Cyc is not comparable to a medical ontology in depth it does posses considerable healthcare terminology and is valuable because it is not limited to healthcare. For the most part, Cyc is not typically used directly for clinical purposes, but can be used in clinical research projects.

LOINC is an ontology of lab result codings that is discussed in Chapter 11.

OpenGALEN and OpenEHR are both attempts to promote open source ontology concepts. Both of the projects have been maturing but some view these as unnecessary additions or alternatives to SNOMED+UMLS. However, they are available under open source licensing terms might make them a better alternative to SNOMED for certain jurisdictions.

One of the largest and fastest growing areas of medical ontologies is *genomic ontologies*. Currently genomic research is conducted outside the normal delivery of care. As typical healthcare providers begin to improve the quality of clinical data that they encode, clinical ontologies like SNOMED CT will be leveraged to bridge normal clinical processes into genomic research areas. As this happens the separation between clinical ontologies and genomic ontologies will begin to fade. For the time being, genomic ontologies are largely separate from clinical ontologies.

There are hundreds of health care, medical, or biological ontologies that we are not covering. Most of them are very focused, like "anatomy of a mouse ontology." A good place to start looking for a particular ontology might be the Open Biological and Biomedical Ontologies Foundry (*http://www.obofoundry.org/*), which has a list of ontologies, or the BioPortal (*http://bioportal.bioontology.org/*) project from the National Center for Biomedical Ontology, which is actually a searchable database of several ontologies.

Sneaky Ontologies

There are several projects that do not sound like ontologies but in fact are. Medical abbreviations are the best example of this. Medical abbreviations are shorthand acronyms or phrases that have well-understood clinical meanings. They can be used when making paper or digital notes without concerns.

Medical abbreviations, especially related to medication instructions, have been well-documented as a significant and dangerous source of medical errors. Many ambiguous medical abbreviations should never be used. There are several lists of these dangerous abbreviations, and a comprehensive list (*http://www.ismp.org/tools/errorproneabbreviations.pdf*) can be found at the Institute for Safe Medication Practices (ISMP). Even after avoiding this list, there is a danger that a clinician will mistype one abbreviation and change it into another.

If these dangers can be avoided, medical abbreviations can save tremendous typing time in an EHR. Modern EHR systems often integrate an abbreviations database that will automatically change medical abbreviations in the longer English descriptions in real time. By allowing the clinician to instantly see what the medical abbreviation that he or she is using actually translates to in real time, medical abbreviations can be made even safer. Moreover, they can dynamically enforce the avoidance of error-prone abbreviations.

There are several efforts to create ontologies that are specifically designed to map from clinical terminology to natural language. Plainlanguage.gov has a section on health literacy (*http://www.plainlanguage.gov/populartopics/health_literacy/index.cfm*) that links to several documents that convert clinical terms into natural language. These dictionaries are the simplest forms of ontologies, mere definitions of terms, with no codes at all. However, these natural language dictionaries can be used to develop PHR interfaces that will contribute substantially to health literacy. Rather than automatically substituting natural language terms for clinical terms, they can simply be added to patient-facing systems. For instance, when a clinical test says "cardiology," that can be replaced with "cardiology (medical treatment of heart problems)."

Ontologies Using APIs

Some ontologies are available as APIs.

The National Provider Identifier database is a database containing most clinicians who can prescribe in the United States. The database is available for download from HHS, and can be searched directly at HHS (*https://nppes.cms.hhs.gov/NPPES/Welcome.do*) or Doc NPI (*http://docnpi.com/*).

You can search for APIs at a general-purpose Programmable Web site (*http://www.programmableweb.com/*). Several ontologies and health data sets are available in the medical and health subsections.

Health.data.gov (*http://www.data.gov/health*) provides a list of data sets that are available for download from the federal government. Although few of the data sets qualify as ontologies, almost all of them are valuable sources for clinical research purposes.

Exercising Ontologies

When actually working with ontologies, you need systems that enable you to store and work with them, integrating them into your clinical IT environment. There are several good open source options known as terminology servers, including Apelon DTS (Distributed Terminology System), which is part of the Open Health Tools (OHT) family of projects. OHT hosts several other important terminology related projects.

The Cancer Biomedical Informatics Grid (CaBIG) (*https://cabig.nci.nih.gov/*) and Informatics for Integrating Biology and the Bedside (i2b2) (*https://www.i2b2.org/i2b2*) are both attempts to leverage clinical and research data for clinical research. Originally, the CaBIG project was exclusively focused on cancer research, but now almost all kinds of clinical research are supported. CaBIG handles research data exchange (usually de-identified data) and have features that help support clinical trials and many other clinical and research processes. i2b2 has always been focused on merging clinical and genomic data sets and clinical ontologies to develop relevant clinical practices.

Protégé (*http://protege.stanford.edu/*) is an open source resource for working with ontologies in the OWL formats.

OpenEHR is a controversial approach to applying knowledge engineering principles to the entire EHR, including things like the user interfaces. You might think of OpenEHR as an ontology for EHR software design. Many health informaticists disagree on the usefulness of OpenEHR. Some believe that HL7 RIM, given its comprehensive nature, is the highest level to which formal clinical knowledge managing needs to go.

CHAPTER 11

Interoperability

The first thing to keep in mind when thinking about interoperability is not a particular standard or technology, but motivations for instituting data exchange. Widescale interoperability has been technically possible for more than 20 years, and major hospitals have had data worth exchanging for at least that long. But as with EHRs, exchanging health data has stalled due to conflicting and backward incentives.

Historically (with a few notable exceptions) most healthcare institutions have found little motivation for interoperability. There is a lot of motivation to *profess* interest in healthcare interoperability, which costs nothing. This creates confusion among those outside the healthcare industry. For example, if the hospital CEO says that interoperability is "critical," why is there no health data being exchanged?

For most clinics and hospitals, making patient data portable makes the patient portable. Why would anyone invest in a technology that makes it easier for patients to migrate to competitors? For any healthcare provider, a patient represents a financial asset that is expensive to replace. And the easy exchange of records lowers one of the main barriers to patients leaving—information about their medical histories. For centuries, a doctor-patient relationship was something very difficult to replicate. Patients understood that their current doctor was familiar with their health story, and moving would mean losing that familiarity. In a world without portable healthcare records, that relationship is priceless to the patient and difficult to rebuild. Changing doctors will still be hard, even when the health record is movable, but it will become a tractable problem.

Similarly, health IT vendors lack motivation to properly support interoperability standards. If the data for a single patient can easily be exported from an EHR, then the data for every patient can also be exported easily. True interoperability means that it is much simpler for one EHR to replace another, and therefore one EHR vendor to be replaced by another. As it stands, without widespread interoperability, it is almost impossible to migrate from one EHR to another. Again, interoperability will not make migration between EHR systems easy, but it will make it possible. EHR vendors know this, and have a similarly mixed motivation regarding interoperability. Most EHR vendors claim that they are interoperable because they provide tools to migrate data into their EHR system. Generally, the motivation for interoperability drops for vendors substantially when they see that it creates a path away from the vendor.

Many EHR vendors charge extra for modules designed to export data, and this fee often becomes a kind of "severance pay" for EHR vendors. When purchasing an EHR, it is critical to request that any modules required for data exchange be included in up-front pricing. Neglecting this often ensures that you have to pay your vendor for the privilege of firing them. Happily, the advent of cheap open source third-party data integration toolkits, such as Mirth Connect (*http://www.mirthcorp.com/products/mirth-connect*), have reduced the impact of this problem.

Some Lessons from Earlier Exchanges

Not all healthcare organizations are disincentivized to interoperate. The exceptions come about when losing a patient is not a real threat. Organizations that sell laboratory services to other healthcare providers are motivated to interoperate because doing so lowers their costs, and they never stand to lose a patient by supporting a data flow. Similarly, many in the safety net community (clinics that charge little to provide care to those in poverty) often struggle to find money to support the patients that they already have. For these types of organizations, the lowered communication costs almost always make any interoperability efforts worthwhile. Obviously, with the complexity caveats covered in Chapter 3, almost all medical billing is done electronically, which counts as a kind of interoperability. Where incentives ensure motivation, healthcare data exchange takes place. The outlook for more generalized healthcare data exchange is more dour.

Originally, an effort to create generalized health information exchanges was called a Community Health Information Network (CHIN). Generally, a CHIN was started by those who recognized the basic value proposition for health information exchange, by funding an organization that made grants to institutions to support exchanges. These efforts, which date back to the late 1980s and early 1990s, generally collapsed once they ran out of funding. Organizations that route health data effectively are expensive to run, and the most common cause of death for such organizations is running out of grant money before achieving the scale needed to self-sustain. Later in the early and late 1990s the same concept was tried again, rebranded as a Regional Health Information Organization (RHIO). Again, the organizations failed when the grant money ran out. The modern term for a RHIO/CHIN is a health information exchange (HIE). All three acronyms—CHIN, RHIO, and HIE—can be used interchangeably. Sadly the postmortem on HIE efforts is just the same. Most HIE efforts go under after the initial funding runs out.

As with other aspects of health IT, it is critical to focus on those organizations that succeeded, rather than those that failed. The best example of a successful HIE in the United States is the Indiana Health Information Exchange. This exchange has been in operation for more than a decade and covers several million patients. Marc Overage, the doctor who runs the exchange, describes three crisis points and how each was overcome (paraphrased from A Brief History of the Indiana Health Information Exchange at *http://indianahimss.org/J_Marc_Overhage_MD-Regenstrief_Institute.pdf*):

- Hospital CIOs argued that ICC competed with individual hospitals' IT strategies to link to physician offices. In the United States, hospitals often affiliate with specialized treatment centers, primary care physicians (family doctors), and so forth, but regulators usually squash these affiliations as anticompetitive and monopolistic unless there is evidence of "clinical integration." As a result, although information exchange between unaffiliated organizations is rare, partnering organizations invest considerable time and capitol in it. General HIE is viewed as competitive with these efforts. The Indiana HIE overcame these protests by emphasizing the reduced costs associated with a city-wide network.

- Hospital CFOs opposed the exchange because they did not see any significant return on investment for their individual organizations. The Indiana HIE showed that the cost of the HIE was equivalent in hard costs to the current operation costs (i.e., faxing and mailing records and lab results). Once it was demonstrated that the HIE's cost would be about the same, any time savings and process improvements become a big deal. These can be harder to measure, and therefore are called soft cost improvements. Soft costs only matter after price parity is demonstrated.

- The HIE had no initial funding, so the Indiana HIE partnered with the Regenstrief Institute for grant funding. (Regenstrief is widely recognized as one of the leading healthcare informatics organizations in the world. It was endowed by an industrialist who made his fortune manufacturing washing machines.) These deep pockets helped ensure that the Indiana HIE would reach the point that it was self-sufficient. Now Indianapolis is one of the few cities in the United States that is largely networked for HIE.

The first two crises demonstrate the lack of motivation among healthcare institutions to support interoperability, and the third demonstrates the difficulty of ensuring a revenue stream.

As we consider which technologies to use for interoperability, we must consider them in the context of the motivations that cause organizations to select them. We must also consider the political implications of the given technology choices. Does the technology require that some central organization exist to provide data routing services? If so, what political influence will that central organization have? If the central organization stores copies of the health records that cross the exchange, the organization will have more influence and capabilities, but will have a harder time building the initial trust to get started. There are many technical issues, such as the data format and security, all with political implications. If you are wise, you will make technology choices that are the least threatening. But assumptions about technical issues can cause enough strife to doom interoperability projects before they begin. Make sure you have made nonthreatening technical choices where you can and then be clear, up front, about your technical plans and strategies to reduce drama.

The New HIE Rules

Thankfully, the fundamental motivation issues that have plagued HIE efforts should soon be things of the past. Meaningful use incentives will ensure that doctors and hospitals will soon be willing to share data with reliable partners, and motivated to work toward generalized healthcare data interchange.

The meaningful use interoperability requirements are trivially simple to achieve in the first year. Only one electronic exchange of health information with one other organization, one time, meets the requirements. But as the requirements for meaningful use advance, doctor's offices and hospitals will not be able meet the requirements without being fully open to HIE based on the standards that we will discuss in this chapter.

Although meaningful use does require specific content standards for HIE, specifically the CCR or the HITSP C32 CCD formats that we will discuss shortly, the standards do not strongly dictate network exchange protocols. This is quite intentional, as there are many cases were existing network protocols are being used to exchange healthcare data, sometimes this is simple secure email attachments. Or perhaps this might be FTP over a VPN, or even Secure Copy (SCP over SSH). Although ONC is deeply investing in two network protocols (IHE and Direct) to replace these ad-hoc networks, they are not being required at this stage. It is obvious that ONC intends to address the content of clinical record exchange at this stage and allow currently existing network methods to count, as long as they meet the basic security requirements of HIPAA. It is also obvious that the network protocols described here will eventually be required. Only the most advanced sites that have been investing in health IT for years are at a place where the content of clinical record exchange is a nonissue. For most sites, this stepping stone approach to HIE makes good sense.

Some of our readers might be looking for the simplest possible network protocol that can meet the meaningful use standards after they already possess a compliant CCR or HITSP C32 file to transfer. The simplest way to accomplish this is probably to use compliant encryption, like advanced encryption standard (AES), encrypt the clinical XML file using a password, email the file to whoever needs it on the other side, and then phone them the password. This is a simple method and it will work for the first year's compliance needs. Long term, you will want to migrate to an approved network protocol, either Direct or IHE. Using phones to transfer passwords will not scale. But before we dive into the content and network protocol standards in question, we need to understand the difference between strong and weak standards.

Strong Standards

Today, even people without a technical orientation have heard of the Domain Name System (DNS), Simple Mail Transfer Protocol (SMTP), File Transfer Protocol (FTP), BitTorrent, and the Hypertext Transfer Protocol (HTTP). These are examples of strong standards. By a strong standard, we mean that one implementation of HTTP, for instance, is always going to work with another implementation of HTTP. The HTTP protocol implementation in Firefox, an open source web browser, will never fail to work with the HTTP protocol implementation in a web server like Apache.

Not all standards are strong, and some technical standards have long been criticized for a weakness that hampers or eviscerates interoperability. A weak standard means that different implementations of a protocol are so different that they are incompatible. HTML (primarily with the Microsoft Internet Explorer implementation) and IPsec (a network encryption protocol) have been historically criticized for this problem. When a standard is weak, different implementations require considerable work to communicate. Sometimes a standard can be so weak that no amount of tweaking can get different implementations to work together.

Generally, standards that are more complex are more difficult to implement correctly in different applications. As a result, simpler standards tend to become strong standards faster than complicated ones.

Interoperability standards are very similar to human languages. Australians, Scots, Irish, Brits, and Americans can understand each other most of the time. If we think of English as a protocol, it is a strong standard. Alternatively if we think of Latin as a protocol, it would be a weak standard, because speakers of dialects that emerged from Latin, such as French and Spanish, cannot automatically understand each other. At one time, Latin might have been a strong standard, but it is certainly not a strong standard now.

Most HIE protocols are weak standards. The only way for any standard to become strong is (a) when users make lots of attempts at communication between different implementations of that standard, and (b) when this pressure drives progress toward standardization. This cross communication must occur until either the standards are changed into something that can be conformed to, or implementations change to match the standard. Either way, the only way for this progress to occur is through lots of attempts at communication. Without any motivation to interoperate, this has not yet happened in healthcare. Meaningful use provides a strong new motivation, and this is now changing. Interoperability workshops are now common among EHR vendors, and several of the protocols we will discuss next have become far stronger than they were even a few years ago.

The problem with many early HIE protocols is that their design encourages individual customization over true standardization. This can happen with real languages, too. For instance, researchers have discovered instances of sign language being reinvented or significantly changing among isolated groups of the deaf. Although communication was occurring, enabled by the new language being built, there was no progress toward the standard. Obviously, for any single group, enabling communication is more important than the long-term strengthening of a standard. If any protocol lends itself to building new languages for fast local communication, rather than enforcing standards, there is typically no progression from a weak standard to a strong standard. Our discussion of older health information protocols will show how they tended to enable new dialects or languages, rather than moving toward standardization. Modern HIE protocols specifically focused on addressing the underlying tension of enabling both flexible communication and enforcing standards to ensure widespread interoperability.

As we discuss the strength of protocols, from a practical perspective, we will refer to the perspective of a "third" implementation. Basically, a standard can be considered strong if, after two different implementations of the protocol succeed in configuring communication, a third implementation can then participate with one of the two original implementations without reconfiguration. If things work from the perspective of the third implementation, the protocol is strong. If the third implementation finds itself shut out, the protocol is weak. Obviously, this heuristic glosses over lots of important technical details, but it is a good rule of thumb. A great real-world example of this, outside health IT, is browser compatibility. Imagine someone creating a new website using Apache, and then, as they built the website, continually testing with the Firefox browser. Here, the third implementation might be Microsoft Internet Explorer. If, after everything works for Firefox, the site also automatically works with Internet Explorer, the underlying protocols involved are strong. This is a good example because a few years ago, this process would regularly break, and now, after the underlying protocols have become stronger, the untested browser tends to work more often in this scenario.

A protocol is only as strong as the conformance of its most popular implementation. Internet Explorer was a poor implementation of web protocols for years, but it was also the most popular. The underlying web standards were perfectly clear; Microsoft had simply ignored and extended them. This creates a substantial power play in the standardization process. Standards bodies that design protocols cannot really make a protocol strong or weak, only protocol implementers can do this. Even subpar standards can become strong protocols when implementers work together well and conform carefully. Mostly, the influence that protocol designers have is to make the path to a strong protocol either an uphill (difficult) or downhill (easy) process. Longer standards with many special cases, leaving room for differences of opinion about details, make conformance an uphill process. Well-engineered implementations of a standard, particularly with open reference implementations that anyone is free to copy or imitate, make conformance a downhill process. Most important, if a standards body does not carefully consider how to handle flexibility, rampant dialectic creation occurs and standardization becomes impossible, no matter what an individual implementation does.

Unfortunately the protocol maturing process in health IT has one significant disadvantage when compared to other IT protocols: all the messages are secrets. Healthcare privacy requirements ensure that implementations of any healthcare protocol are rarely exercised in a public way. In those few cases where there are public simulations of healthcare exchange, using fake, public, or deidentified patient data, tremendous progress is made. But simulations can only go so far in maturing a protocol. This does not mean that healthcare protocols will not mature into strong protocols, but it does ensure that the process takes longer. Of course, there is no question that patient privacy is worth this slowdown, but we must account for it.

Winning Protocols

The protocols that get used in healthcare are not necessarily the best protocols for the job, but the protocols that "won" among implementors.

For billing protocols, which we discuss next, HIPAA determined the winners. Although HIPAA is best known for its privacy rules, it is a general portability law and has a lot to say about billing. HIPAA ultimately required the migration from the National Standard Format (NSF) electronic data interchange format to the ANSI X12 format.

For other health protocols, the winners have generally been chosen by HITSP. HITSP made recommendations to the ONC, which then mandated some of those recommendations as requirements in the meaningful use standards. However, in important cases, ONC has chosen to ignore the final recommendations of HITSP and allowed several standards to meet meaningful use requirements.

The picks made by both of these processes are extremely controversial and still generate considerable debate within the community.

The Billing Protocols

The oldest electronic HIE protocols, being widely adopted in the 1980s, are billing exchange standards based on electronic data interchange (EDI) protocols.

According to legend, EDI dates back to the Berlin airlift. In response to the Western Allies' standardization of money, and knowing that the ruble would crumble in comparison, Stalin closed the Allies' standard supply lines to Berlin. In response the Allies launched an around-the-clock airlift to feed the people of Berlin. But without reliable telephones or radios, they had a problem. They needed to carefully coordinate which ground crews would meet which planes, depending on the planes' contents. Using military teletype, they created a very dense code that could be used to associate each plane (by its tail number) with its time of arrival and contents. Later the automobile industry would adopt technologies inspired by this solution and EDI was fully born.

EDI comes from a time before HTML and XML, a time when a 300-baud modem was fast and expensive. Given those kinds of bandwidth limitations, the same faced during the airlift, it was critical to put as much data as possible into as few characters as possible.

To the untrained eye, NSF and other EDI formats look like intimidating gibberish. Hopefully, our later discussion of HL7 EDI will reduce some of your anxiety about understanding this, but already it should be obvious what the problem with this style of format is: it's hard to tell the difference between correct gibberish and incorrect gibberish. NSF was an important initial medical billing standard, but HIPAA mandates the use of X12.

The basic structure of X12, and many other EDI formats, is:

- Header
- —Patient
  - — —Claim
    - — —Claim component
    - —Claim component
    - —Claim component
  - —Claim
    - — —Claim component
    - —Claim component
    - —etc.
  - —etc.
  - —Patient
  - — —Claim
  - —Claim
  - —etc.
- Footer

The main difference between NSF and X12 is the different delimiters used. X12 also requires more information. X12 looks like this:

```
ISA*00*          *00*          *ZZ*SENDERNAME    *ZZ*RECEIVERNAME
      *110713*1101*U*00501*999999999*0*P*:~
GS*HC*SENDERNAME*RECEIVERNAME*20110713*1101*0000001*X*005010X222~
ST*837*888888*005010X222~
SE*44*888888~
GE*1*999999999~
IEA*1*999999999~
```

This X12 message contains no actual data. What you see are simply the header and footer files for X12. Our purpose here is only to expose you to how X12 data might look. Later we will carefully parse HL7 version 2, which is another EDI format. For now it is enough to note that each "line" starts with a two- or three-letter code that identifies what type of segment it is. Also, in the preceding example we have placed each segment on its own line for readability. The X12 standard does not require this, and regards the tilde (~) as the marker for the end of a segment. That means that this short message could also have been written:

```
ISA*00*         *00*            *ZZ*SENDERNAME   *ZZ*RECEIVERNAME        *110713*1
101*U*00501*999999999*0*P*:~GS*HC*SENDERNAME*RECEIVERNAME*20110713*1101*0000001*
X*005010X222~ST*837*888888*005010X222~SE*44*888888~GE*1*999999999~IEA*1*99999999
9~
```

This is an empty transaction, and a populated transaction could have hundreds more segments just like these. We include these examples only to give you a sense of how X12 looks. If you are working with electronic claims data you will need to become intimately familiar with the standard. Happily, there are many good parsers available for X12 and there are even services online that will tell you if you are generating the standard correctly.

The main reason we bring up billing standards in the interoperability chapter is because billing data is often used to build clinical data. Several different interface engines support X12 conversion, including the open source Mirth project, if you wish to convert useful X12 billing data into clinically acceptable interoperability standards like various forms of HL7. Billing data can, in some cases, be relied on for demographic data, but you should never rely on it directly for clinical data, for reasons we discussed in other chapters.

Generally, X12 implementations are very different, and X12 is a weak standard. CMS does not strongly police adherence to the standard, and payers have strong motivations to maintain nonstandard implementations, as described in Chapter 3. As you generate or parse X12 files, remember that they are typically generated to suite a particular exchange relationship. That relationship really is the standard for the file, and the X12 standard is just the inspiration for that local standard.

HL7 Version 2

Another tried and true HIE protocol is HL7, which stands for Health Layer 7. In the Open Systems Interconnection (OSI) model of network protocols, layer seven was the top, application layer. So the 7 is simply a reference to HL7's existence as a network protocol. HL7 is developed by the Health Layer Seven International standards body.

HL7 is a protocol designed for signaling changes to a patient's record using short messages. When a single detail of a patient's record changes, that change can usually be sent to another health information system using an HL7 message.

HL7 is intended to be implemented on top of other networking protocols, and indeed everything from direct TCP/IP (the low-level Internet protocol) or HTTP/FTP are used to deliver HL7 messages.

Early versions of HL7 are densely formatted EDI-style messages. Currently variations of the second version of HL7 are in widespread use. HL7 v1.x was used so briefly that almost no ongoing use occurs. HL7 versions are not compatible between major revisions, so no 2.x version is compatible with any 3.x version. HL7 versions are intended to be backward compatible with minor version numbers, so a message sent by a 2.1 compatible system should be fully parsable by a 2.2 compliant implementation, and so on. In reality, version issues are very commonly the bane of an HL7 implementer's existence. Small changes between versions often cause parsing problems and are frequently the source of errors.

You will probably see lots of late version 2 version streams (2.5,2.6, 2.7, etc.). These streams are usually represented in the EDI-style format we are discussing here, but it is possible to represent them in XML. The EDI format is more difficult and counterintuitive for modern IT professionals, so we will skip version 2 XML representations. If you can understand the more common, EDI-based variations of HL7 v2.x, you will find the XML representations a simple transition.

Ringholm, a company that offers training in HL7 across Europe, has an excellent white paper (*http://www.ringholm.de/docs/04300_en.htm*) that shows the same information encoded in several versions of HL7. Because it is Creative Commons licensed, it serves as an excellent framework to discuss variations of HL7, and you can and should reuse these examples as you try to spread understanding of HL7 in your own organization.

Version 2.x of the protocol works like so:

```
MSH|^~\&|GHH LAB|ELAB-3|GHH OE|BLDG4|200202150930||ORU^R01|CNTRL-3456|P|2.4<cr>
PID|||555-44-4444||EVERYWOMAN^EVE^E^^^L|JONES|19620320|F|||153 FERNWOOD DR.^
^STATESVILLE^OH^35292||(206)3345232|(206)752-121||||AC555444444||67-A4335^OH^200
30520<cr>
OBR|1|845439^GHH OE|1045813^GHH LAB|15545^GLUCOSE|||200202150730|||||||||| 555-55-
5555^PRIMARY^PATRICIA P^^^^MD^^|||||||||F||||||444-44-4444^HIPPOCRATES^HOWARD H^
^^^MD<cr>
OBX|1|SN|1554-5^GLUCOSE^POST 12H CFST:MCNC:PT:SER/PLAS:QN||^182|mg/dl|70_105|H|||
F<cr>
```

If you have a background in IT, the next paragraphs will probably seem pretty basic, but if you have a healthcare background, now is a good time to talk a bit about parsing. Otherwise, the preceding example is simply too unsettling for our clinical readers to consider further.

Computers are good at representing text, but not good at understanding what the text means. Computers are also good at breaking text up into component parts, which can make it easier for them to understand what certain pieces of information are. The computational process of breaking up text into smaller parts is called *parsing*. Symbols that are intentionally inserted into text to make them parsable by computers are called *markup*.

The web revolution occurred, in great part based on two innovations that Tim Berners-Lee inserted into HTML: the first was hypertext links, and the second was human readable markup (an innovation borrowed from an earlier standard called SGML). HTML was the first popular markup format that was clearly intended to be both parsable by software (i.e., your browser) and readable by humans. What Berners-Lee realized was that modern networking systems could move enough data that he no longer needed as a design goal to make transmitted text markup as compact as possible. We no longer needed to account for the bandwidth limitations of a 300-baud modem, or the military teletype used in the Berlin airlift. XML was developed to be a generalizable implementation of this idea that HTML had popularized.

As tools for using XML proliferated, technologists in many fields realized that all information, not just web pages, could be marked up in a way that was both computer parsable and human readable. A nontechnical reader (we can all remember what it was like to be a nontechnical reader) might have a sinking feeling in her stomach when reading the gibberish in our example HL7 message. XML makes messages like these much easier and less intimidating to read, and although currently this type of unintelligible EDI is very common, the industry is moving toward XML.

In short, if you are a nontechnical reader, let us state what our technical readers already know: in health IT, XML is your friend. Tim Berners-Lee was knighted for his contributions to the World Wide Web, and with insights like these, this should bolster our faith in the British monarchy.

With that in mind, we can now begin to take apart the previous HL7 message in the way that the computer would read it. This manual parsing process will help us understand how HL7 v2, as well as earlier EDI standards like X12 and NSF, are used. Parsing is simply the breaking apart of the message into smaller parts that have specific meanings. So to start, we break the message apart starting with the highest level possible, *segments*. Segments are separated by the symbol for a carriage return, <cr>. Basically, that is the same thing as pressing the Enter or Return key on your keyboard. So the segments are like paragraphs in writing, separated by explicitly moving to the next line. To make that clearer, we include the symbol <cr> at the end of the segments. Looking at the message and noting the locations of the <cr> symbols, we can now easily see that the first segment is:

```
MSH|^~\&|GHH LAB|ELAB-3|GHH OE|BLDG4|200202150930||ORU^R01|CNTRL-3456|P|2.4<cr>
```

This process of splitting a large text string into several smaller ones, based on a character or series of characters, is a specific kind of markup called *delimiting*. The character or string of characters that we use to split the text into smaller parts is called the *delimiter*. A delimiter is just a particular case of markup.

The first segment in HL7 is the message header. It gives general information about the whole message. The next level to parse is the *field*. Fields are separated by the | (vertical bar) symbol. So if we split and number the fields of this segment we get:

```
1 = MSH
2 = ^~\&
3 = GHH LAB
```

```
4 = ELAB-3
5 = GHH OE
6 = BLDG4
7 = 200202150930
8 = blank field!!
9 = ORU^R01
10 = CNTRL-3456
11 = P
12 = 2.4
```

Now we start to get to the underlying meaning from the parsing (which is the whole point of any markup). The HL7 standard says that the first field of any segment tells you what kind of segment it is. This is an MSH segment, which stands for message header. The name of each segment is always three letters long, making the vertical bar character always the fourth character. This makes it very simple to determine what the purpose of each segment is.

From there, we can look up the segment type MSH in the HL7 v2 standard to determine what all of the other fields mean:

```
1 = Segment Type = MSH
2 = Field Separator = ^~\&
3 = Sending Application = GHH LAB
4 = Sending Facility = ELAB-3
5 = Receiving Application = GHH OE
6 = Receiving Facility = BLDG4
7 = Date/Time of message = 200202150930
8 = blank field!!
9 = Message Type = ORU^R01
10 = Message Control ID = CNTRL-3456
11 = Message Processing ID = P
12 = Message Version = 2.4
```

The MSH or message header segment tells us what segments are going to follow in the rest of the message. It also gives us important information about how the message is encoded. Theoretically, a message like this could be sent, and an implementation could read the information in the header and automatically know how to process the request. In reality, almost every message type in every message stream must be carefully examined to ensure that its contents are correct, no matter what the MSH segment advertises. As we'll see soon, implementations do not always use the standard properly.

The second field of the MSH header notes the characters that will be used to further mark up each field. These are generally the same in every HL7v2 message, and have the following meaning:

^ = *component separator*
   (a component is what a field splits into)

~ = *repetition separator*
   (some fields repeat, and this character separates instances of the same field)

\ = *the escape character*
   (explained later)

& = *subcomponent separator*
   (components can have parts, too; yes, the standard is that brutal)

Sometimes you need to use one of the delimiter fields in the actual text of a message, (something like "Johnson & Johnson"). The escape character tells an implementation when a character should really be itself, and not treated as a delimiter. Sadly, you should not assume that your HL7 implementation or your partners understand how to use the escape character. Strange errors result when this does not work properly. Remember that HL7 is a point-to-point communications protocol and that usually, you will not have the privilege of controlling both sides of the conversation. This example, for instance, is a lab result being received as the result of a lab request. Even if your HL7 implementation properly supports escape characters, if your lab provider does not, your messages could be mangled. Most importantly, messages could get mangled at some future point in time, because, for instance, of a new patient name. (It is not without irony that we can list "O'Reilly" as precisely the type of name that can cause serious errors in HL7 parsing, thanks to the apostrophe in the name).

Next comes the sender and receiver data:

   3 = Sending Application = GHH LAB
   4 = Sending Facility = ELAB-3
   5 = Receiving Application = GHH OE
   6 = Receiving Facility = BLDG4

While this seems simple, it can be difficult because of the different ways there are to arrange the information. For instance, should Sending Application be the name of the software implementing HL7? Or should it be the server running the application? Or perhaps both? Should a facility (in Sending Facility and Receiving Facility) mean the name of the chain of hospitals that a lab is associated with, the name of the hospital, the name of the lab department within the hospital, or the names of all three?

These things matter more and more as you develop multiple HL7 streams with different clinical partners. (A stream just refers to all the messages regularly moving back and forth as a whole between two institutions. Another name for this is channel.) Eventually, workflow logic will start to rely heavily on the contents of these fields, and decisions made when the first HL7 streams were created will seem short-sighted. However, once a stream of HL7 messages is stable, it is difficult and often dangerous to modify their operation. Most organizations choose to live with many decisions made when the stream was already created.

Date and time of the message is largely self-explanatory, but it is very possible to mess this up. Systems might decide to time stamp the creation of the order, the creation of the sample, the receipt of the lab order, the time the lab was created, or the time and date that the message was sent. The latter is actually the correct value according to the standard.

```
7 = Date/Time of message = 200202150930
```

Next, we have the message type. This will determine, generally, what type of segments will be included in the rest of the message. This field has two components. The first component is ORU, which means that this is the response to a lab order, with the lab results. This code implies that you will find the OBR and OBX segments, which contain the actual lab result data as well as PID, which should contain patient data. The R01 following the ORU means that this is an unsolicited transmission. That sounds strange, but what it really means is that this message was not sent as a direct result of some other message. It was sent because the lab result was completed.

```
9 = Message Type = ORU^R01
```

The next segment is the message control ID, which is the code that uniquely identifies this message from every other message. As you can see it is possible and common to put some other information in this field that could be parsed out and have some purpose. Here, the content is divided by the hyphen (-), and to the right is an ID. Very often, this ID field includes some reference to another message ID, which is the mechanism by which messages are linked. For instance, if a lab request is made in one message, the ID field of the lab result message might include the message ID of the lab request message.

This message control ID should be unique on a per-sender basis. That is, you should never get the same message control ID twice from the same sender, but don't count on it. A good HL7 engine will take the Message Control ID + Sender ID into account when considering message uniqueness, but will detect both identical resends of the same message, and reuse of the same IDs in new messages. Systems implementing HL7 will often define the Message Control ID on some other datapoint that they believe ensures uniqueness, but it actually does not ensure uniqueness. Again, this is an issue that a receiving HL7 engine can handle, assuming it is high quality.

```
10 = Message Control ID = CNTRL-3456
```

The 11th slot is Message Processing ID. Sometimes, you need to mark a message as a test message, or need to make a message as an example. As you set up and debug your second or later HL7 message stream, this field will be critical for your testing purposes. You might need to support testing and production data on the same HL7 channel and this is field is how you will do that.

```
11 = Message Processing ID = P
```

The value of P here indicates that this message is a production message, containing real data to act on. Generally you can trust that messages with a P here should be treated as production messages. But you should not presume that messages without a P are not production messages. For instance, if a message was dropped and needs to be re-sent, an implementation might send the second message with an R for "restore from archive."

The last slot in this example message (but not in the standard for the MSH segment) is the HL7 version that the message uses. This is a relatively old version, 2.4, which still sees wide use.

```
12 = Message Version = 2.4
```

This brings us to the `<cr>` symbol and therefore the end of this segment. We will not go into this level of detail for the following segments. Generally, to parse a segment you need to understand what the HL7 standard says should be in the segment, as well as what data you are actually getting. Though the fields for each segment are different, the process of splitting and categorizing the fields will be identical to what we did here with the MSH segment.

For the most part, you need to ensure that every potential class of HL7 message you receive will be parsed correctly. We say "class" here, because sometimes, an implementation will send messages that advertise to be of the same message type, but are in fact operating very differently.

For instance, in the example message, the segments after the MSH are PID (Patient Identification), OBX (Observation Request), and OBR (Observation). Generally, observation request segments detail what was ordered, while observation segments detail the results of the tests. However, many lab requests are for panels of labs, which means that one request is actually a bundling of several other requests. Some implementations might choose to use the OBX segment to detail the panel, and add information regarding the component tests in several different OBR segments. Another implementation might choose to have several OBX segments detailing the component tests, and have a matching OBR for each test, all in the same HL7 message. Other implementations might choose to create entirely separate HL7 messages, as though there was no panel bundling in the order at all.

Several critical fields in the OBX segment should be mentioned. The third field of OBX, or OBX-3, is the name of the test being done. The HL7 standard allows locally defined values in this field, but unless you have a very good reason not to (and you probably don't) you should be using Logical Observation Identifiers Names and Codes (LOINC) values in this field. LOINC was developed by the Regenstrief Institute (the same one we discussed earlier) in 1994 to help ensure that lab results coming from different lab providers would be comparable. Without it, there is no way to ensure interoperability of the lab data that is transferred using HL7. If you have a new HL7 project, start right off using LOINC and save yourself the painful process of migrating data from local codes to LOINC later. If you are not using LOINC, start doing so and begin the painful process of migrating data from local codes to LOINC. Thankfully, Regenstrief released a second tool to help with the process of mapping local codes to LOINC. The tool is called RELMA, which aptly stands for Regenstrief LOINC Mapping Assistant.

The second critical field in OBX is field five, which contains the data type of the observed value. This should be a SNOMED CT code. SNOMED CT is extensively described in the Chapter 10.

The most substantial problem with HL7 v 2.x, like the billing EDI formats, is its capacity to support local communication at the expense of standardization. As we mentioned in the beginning of the chapter, a standard's capacity to build new dialects of itself hinders widespread interoperability. HL7 v 2.x has two main mechanisms that lead to a lack of standardization.

First, because it is simple to place more data at the end of a given line, implementers often "extend" the standard by simply placing more data they want at the end of what should be a standardized segment. Of course, because this ignores the standard, there is no way that a third implementation can account for this kind of variation.

The second destandardization mechanism is the Z segment. Z segments are segments that are defined by the user. Like all segments, Z segments must begin with a three-letter name. However, HL7 allows that if a name begins with a Z, it can be entirely user defined. Usually, a Z segment is an indication of a workaround that was the result of a historical issue with HL7 v2, or the result of ignorance or laziness on the part of the implementer (or both).

HL7 v2 is an expansive standard that can now be used to automate the majority of common health information systems communications, at least those that respond well to a message-based approach. For instance, if you want to export a summary of a patient's record, HL7 v2 cannot really help. A summary of a patient's record includes lots of divergent information all bundled together, but an HL7 message speaks to one single clinical datapoint at a time.

HL7 was not always so expansive. Version 1 of HL7 was so short lived that it might as well be considered a beta, making early 2.x versions the first reliable HL7 messaging system. At that time, having Z segments was a critical part of ensuring that HL7 could meet unexpected clinical use-cases. Streams of HL7 that continue to use Z segments extensively come with a stiff penalty. Late versions of HL7 2.x carefully support most valid use-cases for system-to-system messaging in health IT. Best practices when setting up new HL7 channels include completely forbidding HL7 Z segments until it is proven that no other predefined segment type can work. This ensures that at least new implementations of HL7 v2 can contribute to a semantically interoperable HIE process. Because Z segments are custom containers, it is not possible to rely on their contents semantically in any kind of formulaic way.

It would be wonderful if we could update all low-version HL7 2.x streams to later version streams. It would be wonderful if we could update all of the old-school vertical bar syntax HL7 to XML. But the investment required to do that rarely pays off. However, upgrading the stream version, or even, in some cases, downgrading the stream version is a common practice. Usually this is because old versions no longer work for some reason. Upgrading a working stream is rarely worth it, but when streams break, often an upgrade is the only way to restore functionality. Often, software upgrades in other parts of a health IT infrastructure will force an upgrade to a new HL7 version.

Besides billing data, HL7 v2.x traffic is by far the most common form of interoperability. But this section was intended to both give you an introduction into the format and to warn you of the difficulties involved in typical HL7 stream implementations. Most summaries of HL7, especially those released by the HL7 consortium, merely introduce the format, without properly setting expectations. No health IT expert we are aware of would contradict the statement that HL7 interoperability is difficult and can blind-side those who are unfamiliar with the domain. We hope that your environment won't have all the problems we've mentioned, but in reality, we have probably not prepared you for the exceptions and difficulties that you will experience.

Moreover, any HL7 channel requires ongoing maintenance and monitoring. We have given several examples of how new data (i.e., the first time that a last name with an apostrophe, such as "O'Reilly," goes through the system) can have unintended consequences. But servers and networking equipment frequently just die. There are many reasons why your stream could be down or contain errors. Once a new stream of HL7 has stabilized, it will be very reliable, except when it isn't. It is important that someone be watching to catch and repair mistakes quickly. Once a clinical workflow becomes deeply reliant on an HL7 stream, clinicians will begin to assume that the data will always appear on time.

We know of at least one person who was killed because an interface was down. In this case, the clinician misinterpreted the signal in the EHR UI that the interface was down to mean that no lab result existed. The lab result did exist and required immediate attention. A young child died as the result of the error. When one anecdote like this exists, it is reasonable to assume that this type of problem has killed or injured many more people. This is one example of the new class of medical errors that are the result of the addition of health IT systems. Many healthcare shops cannot afford the luxury of redundant servers, and most HL7 streams rely on a chain of single servers. This makes automated log and uptime monitoring critical to the safe deployment of HL7 streams. Also be aware that the logs from interface engines could often contain HIPAA-covered data, and must be protected accordingly. No HL7 interface engine infrastructure should be considered without a monitoring solution. There have been many reports of immature HL7 products that do not properly support logging and monitoring, so this should be part of your acquisition requirements.

There are basically two different ways to work with HL7. First, most mature health IT software, especially from larger vendors, has integrated HL7 functionality. Most of the suffering from HL7 v2.x comes from these implementations. A whole health IT sub-industry exists specifically to solve the problem of repairing, modifying, and rerouting streams of HL7 v2.x data. Software that does this is typically called an *integration engine*. Fortunately, some excellent HL7 integration engines are available. There are several competent vendors of interface engines, including InterfaceWare, and Intersystems with its Ensemble product. Oracle and Microsoft also offer EDI interfacing engines, but they are often more general toolkits that are underpowered for healthcare. They will work, but they will require more sweat.

We already mentioned an open source interface engine called Mirth Connect. Mirth Connect was the first of several open source interoperability products from MirthCorp, and as a result is still often referred to as just "Mirth." Mirth is by far the most popular open source project in healthcare, because it can be easily paired with both proprietary and open source health IT systems, including EHRs and lab information systems (LIS). In many ways Mirth is comparable to the Apache web server: it runs on multiple platforms, is the dominant open source project in its space, and is the dominant product in its category. Just like there are reasons to not use Apache in certain environments, there are reasons not to use Mirth. Like Apache, however, most people start with Mirth, and then discard it only when their use case becomes non-general.

Interface consulting, from MirthCorp or a reliable proprietary interface engine company, is generally worthwhile. Developing an HL7 channel is a lot like flying a plane. Just moving around in the air is simple because airplanes are very stable and there is little to run into, but takeoff and landing are very difficult, experience and training matter a lot, and mistakes are costly. For HL7, creating and validating a new stream of HL7 data is very complicated, but once that work is done, maintaining a stream is a much easier, if constant, task. Usually, it is worth the money to hire experienced HL7 consultants, but frequently no money is set aside for non-core health IT projects. If you have more than one internal health IT system, or you know you need to communicate with organizations in a message-oriented fashion, you need to budget either time or money to solve the problem with an HL7 engine of some kind.

First-Generation and Second-Generation HIEs

The technical approaches taken by RHIOs and HIEs historically have been to position themselves as a kind of HL7 v2 hub. HL7 v2 is deeply message oriented, and those messages are designed to be A→B style messages, going from one party to another party. However, you could always have that message go to from one party to a second party through a third party. For the most part, HIE technical designs have focused on being that third party.

This man-in-the-middle model, which is shared by medical claims clearinghouses using the X12 standard, has some pretty substantial limitations. The most important of these is that the network itself is not capable of summarizing the current healthcare status of a patient. Instead, all the HIE network has is a history of a patient's transactions.

Second-generation HIE efforts are all designed to address this limitation by improving the content of the message, and improving the protocols used to deliver the messages. First we will talk about the options to improve clinical message contents.

Continuity of Care Record

The CCR is a standard developed by ASTM International and supported by the American Academy of Family Physicians. ASTM used to stand for American Society for Testing and Materials, and they saw no reason to give up a familiar abbreviation just to be an international organization. Now they go by the name ASTM followed by the reassuring "International."

CCR work was begun in 2003 and was approved by ASTM in 2005. Its core philosophy was a direct reaction to the architectural problems with HL7 2.x. HL7 2.x, which we just covered, is a messaging protocol between computer systems. It was never intended to be human readable, and more important, there is no way that a single HL7 2.x message can summarize the healthcare of a patient.

HL7 2.x was designed to represent what is happening to a patient right now, and CCR was designed to be a summary of everything that has happened to a patient up till now. In many ways, CCR was the first healthcare standard to embrace both the expressive power and the human readability promised by the XML format. Like HL7, CCR can be thought of in terms of messages, but with a very different style. CCR is a really big message saying everything (summary is the term used most often) and HL7 v2 is a series of really small messages that say just what recently happened. Theoretically, the history of all small HL7 v2 messages together could describe everything known about a patient, but practically that would never work—most of the time only a small subset of message types are actually transferred using HL7 v2 (usually just lab results).

In response to the release and popularity of CCR, the HL7 standards body began creating a new standard, called the Continuity of Care Document (CCD) that would be an extension of the CCR, and also embrace the new Clinical Document Architecture (CDA) that HL7 was developing as part of HL7 v3. HL7 had been developing CDA, which was an XML-document based approach to summary documents, for several years. Compliance with the CDA and HL7 RIM (explained in the next section) ensured that CCD was a much more capable standard, but this capacity came at the expense of human readability.

Although CCD was an technically an extension of CCR, the standards quickly became fierce competitors. The health IT industry quickly drew lines with small vendors (who preferred standards that were simpler to implement) typically siding with CCR and large vendors (experienced in the HL7 development process) choosing CCD. Ultimately HITSP would settle on the HL7 standards of CCD/CDA/RIM over CCR in its recommendations to ONC for the standards required in meaningful use.

Dr. David Kibbe is an MD who has focused on health IT for years. Dr. Kibbe was the founding director of the Center for Health Information Technology (*http://www.cen terforhit.org/*) for the American Academy of Family Physicians (AAFP). Dr. Kibbe and the AAFP have advocated for simplicity in healthcare technology for years. This makes sense, because while the AMA represents all doctors, the AAFP represents primary care physicians with the smallest budgets, often operating with the most constrained resources. This is the community of doctors most vulnerable to health IT failures and most central to the success of the meaningful use program. Dr. Kibbe has been a long-time supporter of the CCR standard and advised HL7 to keep it simple in their development of the CCD standard, advice they largely ignored.

After HITSP announce its exclusive support for HL7 CCD over CCR, Kibbe wrote in a famous blog post (*http://e-caremanagement.com/untangling-the-electronic-health -data-exchange/*) saying:

> It is the epitome of a top-down, large established player-controlled, and anti-competitive juggernaut in which a "one size fits all" paradigm has been promoted and lobbied for. In this case, HITSP has "selected" the CCD and not the CCR standard, despite the market forces that seem to be continuing the use of the CCR standard. This is simply stupid and likely will turn out to be futile.

Kibbe had a point. The CCR is a much cleaner and simpler protocol to implement and to read than the CCD. The CCD does more and has more features, but is much more complex and difficult to work with as a result. Generally, committees that evaluate technological issues pick solutions that are complex, because only complex solutions have enough features to make most of the committee happy. It looks like this is precisely what HITSP did (*http://publicaa.ansi.org/sites/apdl/hitspadmin/Matrices/HITSP_09_N _451.pdf*).

Conversely, the marketplace tends to pick the simplest tool that might get the job done, preferring speed and simplicity over more comprehensive and unwieldy solutions. The most famous example of this was the success of the first iPhone from Apple. The first iPhone was controversial in the industry for lacking so many features that other smart-phones at the time supported, including simple cut-and-paste. The market, however, amply rewarded the simple iPhone approach, and eventually Apple added missing features, like cut-and-paste. This marketplace trend is generally called a *disruptive innovation* after a term coined by Clayton M. Christensen and explained in the book *Innovators Dilemma*. (Christensen also authored a book about the general implications for the concept in healthcare, called the *Innovators Prescription*, which is worth reading).

As evidence for this preference in the marketplace; Microsoft HealthVault chose to accept both CCR and CCD, but Google Health chose only to accept a limited subset of the CCR document as acceptable for clinical information input.

After the HITSP recommended HL7 CDA/CDD, it looked like CCR was a dead format. The final rule for meaningful use changed that. In the response to comments, the protocol section of the final rule states:

> We adopted both the CCR and CCD as patient summary record standards.

> We adopted both standards for a few reasons. First, we are aware, contrary to some commenters' statements, that a significant segment of the HIT industry still uses the CCR patient summary record standard and that some health care providers prefer the CCR over the CCD. For this reason, we did not want to mandate, at such an early stage, that

all of these early adopters adopt a different summary record standard for the purposes of meaningful use Stage 1, given that electronic HIE is not required. Second, we understand that in some circumstances the CCR is easier, faster, and requires fewer resources to implement than the CCD. We have therefore concluded that it was appropriate to adopt the CCR standard for patient summary records in this initial set of standards. Finally, we believe that at the present time, each standard could equally be used to satisfy the requirements of meaningful use Stage 1.

No matter whether you agree with Kibbe and the AAFP and prefer the simple and elegant approach of CCR, or agree with HITSP and HL7 and prefer the functionality offered by CCD, the key phrases to read from this notice are "both" and "at the present time."

This means that ONC is not committing to both the CCR and the CCD forever. Future revisions of the meaningful use standard may select one of the standards exclusively, or even a third patient summary standard as yet unknown. However, for the present time, supporting both standards is the order of the day. To be meaningfully use-certified, an EHR must support both CCR and CCD formats. For the most part, this means that clinical users do not have to worry about the debate, as both formats will just work in their systems. But the underlying differences between the standards are critical for health IT professionals to understand.

Happily, XML itself provides a partial solution to the problem of supporting both CCR and CCD. Extensible Stylesheet Language Transformations (XSLT) is a declarative language that translates XML documents into other formats, including other XML documents. Converting CCR into CCD using XSLT is a well-understood process. It is not possible to always convert all of the information in a CCD document to CCR since some CCD features are not supported in CCR, but to the degree that it is possible, XSLT can do it.

Even aside from the CCR/CCD debate, XSLT is a critical technology for patient care summary documents, because it is the preferred way to translate a CCR or CCD document into a paper document or an HTML web page. Meaningful use requires that patients have access to CCR or CCD documents and paper versions of those same summaries. Using XSLT, it is possible to meet both requirements easily using only CCR or CCD. The fact that XSLT is itself actually written in XML leads us to reiterate: In health IT, XML is your friend.

HL7 v3, RIM, CDA, CDD, and HITSP C32

HL7 version 3 should probably be considered a completely different standard from version 2, and really merits a different name, rather than merely a new version number. Version 3 is capable of replicating the message-oriented use case of version 2 HL7, but it is also capable of far more. In reality, version 3 of HL7 is not one standard at all, but a family of standards that are used for different purposes. We have already mentioned that CCD and the underlying CDA are part of HL7 v3.

The heart of HL7 v3 is the Reference Implementation Model (RIM). The HL7 3 RIM is an information model that generally describes how entities, who play roles, can act on other entities over time. If that sounds pie-in-the-sky abstract, it is only because it is. RIM is not actually healthcare-specific, but rather a high-level way of establishing fundamental relationships. RIM is a controversial idea. Some people regard RIM as too abstract and to distant from real life to be useful. Others believe that this super-high-level model is critical for ensuring that very different healthcare standards still share the same underlying notions.

There are only six basic object types in the RIM model. First are Acts, Roles, and Entities, which can be connected by ActRelationship (between acts), Participation (connections between Entities and Acts, which have Roles), and RoleLink (between roles). The backbone of RIM is simply that everything being modeled is *an Entity in a Role that is Participating in an Act*.

Everything else in RIM is either some kind of extension of or modifier for one of the basic object types. The whole notion of acts lends the model a notion of time. Acts can have states that happen during, after, or before, or even things that happen if the act fails to take place. People are a kind of entity, and can play different roles in different acts. We can imagine how simple healthcare concepts play out under this very basic model:

> Today (the time modifier for an act) Nurse (a role) Susan (a person, which is an entity) gives a shot to (an act) patient (a role) Tom. Tom is also a doctor (a role) and tomorrow (a time modifier for an act) will place a Band-Aid (an act) on Susan (a person), who is a patient (role) at that time.

RIM is flexible: it can also model a children's cartoon.

> Tom (cat, which is an entity) is the hunter (role) and chases (an act) Jerry (mouse, which is an entity), the prey (a role) today (time modifier). Before (time modifier) Tom catches (an act) Jerry (a mouse), a dog (an entity) begins to hunt (act) Tom (entity), who is now the prey (role).

We asked Dr. Peter Hendler, who works with RIM extensively at Kaiser Permanente to give us a real-world example of RIM in action:

> An Aspirin tab is in the role of "Administered Substance" Participating in an Act of Substance Administration. In the same Act. An Entity person is in the role of subject also Participating in the same act of Substance Administration. Normally a Prescription is written like this:
>
>> Prednisone 5mg, dispense 100, Refills 2
>> Take one pill a day by mouth.
>
> This, in the RIM, consists of two acts. The first act of dispensing 100 pills in a bottle is a Supply Act. The second act is the Substance Administration where one a day is taken by mouth.
>
> The two acts are related by an Act Relationship. An Entity person in the Role of the pharmacist participates in the Supply Act. The Participants of the Substance Administration are the same.

The real value of RIM is that it allows you to talk about these basic concepts, and extensions of them, carefully. For instance, RIM handles the minutiae of how all of these objects should be given IDs. Those IDs are then used extensively inside XML standards, and therefore XML documents that are RIM-based.

From that simple basis, the real work of HL7 begins. Most of the guts of the HL7 process are constraining RIM. The process for these constraints builds the limitations inherent in the world that HL7 wants to model, which is healthcare. Healthcare is different, in some cases, from cartoons, which would require different constraints. Constraints enable RIM to be specified in a manner that is appropriate for clinical messages (similar to HL7 v2) in some cases, and clinical documents in others. Because clinical constraints are so common among the goals of HL7, there is a great deal of time spent ensuring that constraints are reusable.

For the most part, all of this is totally irrelevant to the end user and administrator of health IT technology that leverages HL7 v3, so we are glossing over a tremendous amount of detail. Most of that detail is important only to health IT software developers who would like to get RIM to be constrained in other interesting ways.

For everyone else it is enough to know that the process by which RIM becomes useful is by constraints and that at the end of this "constraining" process, out pop XML schemas. An XML schema is an XML document that defines how other XML documents should behave. RIM is constrained into several different XML schemas that have different purposes, but the most important of these for interoperability is the previously mentioned CDA.

CDA provides a high-level definition of how clinical documents should look. It has three "levels." All three can be validated by the same XML schema. *Validation* is a process where an XML validation program (of which there are many) compares an XML file to an XML schema to determine whether the file is compliant with the schema.

The three levels for CDA implement what HL7 calls incremental semantic interoperability. This is shorthand for saying that low levels of CDA are not semantically interoperable, and higher levels are. Low levels of CDA are simple to make, high levels are hard to make. Specifically:

- Level 1 CDA compliance is met by placing clinical free text or a graphical image inside an XML file. The XML contains only the image or text and as much metadata regarding that text as possible. This means, of course, that you can scan in paper records as digital images and be CDA Level 1 compliant.
- Level 2 CDA compliance supports the same digital content, but requires that the clinical content be marked up in a fashion surprisingly similar to HTML.
- Level 3 CDA compliance supports digital content, but requires that the clinical markup be semantically coded using healthcare code sets such as LOINC or SNOMED CT.

This is the point where it gets pretty interesting. Our main interest in the CDA is to help us move data around to give a complete snapshot of a given patient. The preferred way to that is to further constrain the contents of a CDA document into a CCD, so how should that happen? By emulating the contents of a CCR to define the contents of a CDA document. This means that a CCD is just RIM, constrained all the way down to what was already in a CCR. But all of those constraints mean that CCD XML documents are capable of encoding a great deal more content than a CCR. Most importantly, a CCR is really only capable of being one kind of clinical document, a summary of a patient's health record, whereas a CCD is capable of being other kinds of clinical documents, like discharge summaries.

The HL7 standards process intentionally left the majority of the contents of a CCD document as optional, so you can have a CCD that is a complete summary of the patient's health record from birth, or a document that has only the basic demographics of a patient—both are equally valid.

HITSP addressed this by adding further constraints for the elements of a CCD that are required for interoperability efforts. The name of the this standard is HITSP C32, or just C32 for short.

Figure 11-1 illustrates the relationships between the various HL7 standards.

The actual experience of working directly with HITSP C32 can be daunting. For our readers who are somewhat familiar with XML, HITSP C32 ends up being relatively attribute heavy. These attributes are the method for linking all the way back to RIM, so they are important, but ugly. The structure of the XML is also somewhat inconsistent. Sometimes, the designers of the schema seem to prefer using XML as a kind of tree structure, and other times, they seem to prefer using XML as a list. Both approaches to encoding XML are fine, but it can be difficult to work with one XML schema that alternates between the two as heavily as HITSP C32 does. The main benefit of XML, usually, is that it makes life simpler, and some of these design decisions serve to take away from that benefit. For the reader, our advice is simple. If you are going to be working directly with these XML files, prepare to make an investment in time to understand the complexities involved. We wish we could say that most of our readers will not need to work directly with the files, but because almost all of these standards are weak, it is inevitable that individual files will need to be frequently studied to debug new instances of data exchange. Eventually, software, either in the IHE/Direct stack or in the EHR stack, will learn to hide you from these complexities, but for now, expect some road bumps. Still, these formats are XML, and XML provides strong generalized tools to ensure a modicum of standard compliance.

All of these standards end up being encoded in XML schemas that can be used by XML validation software to determine whether a given XML file is, in fact, acting properly. Happily, you do not need to download all of these schemas or find XML validation software to determine whether a given XML file is compliant with these standards. The National Institute of Standards and Technology (NIST) makes a web service available

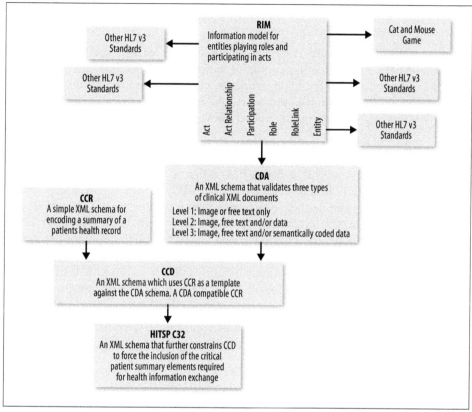

Figure 11-1. HL7 standards

that will test any XML file for compliance. As long as your EHR or other health IT software can generate attempts at C32-compliant XML without real patient data inside (i.e., using dummy data), you can upload that file to the CDA Guideline Validation site (*http://xreg2.nist.gov/cda-validation/validation.html*) and have NIST test to see that your implementation is standards compliant. This validation tool can test C32 compliance, which automatically checks to make sure that the document is also CCD and CDA compliant. The service can also check to ensure that other types of CDA documents are compliant, such as those required by IHE, which we will talk about next. Before you upload your files to NIST for compliance testing, be sure to de-identify any real patient data inside.

The IHE Protocol

IHE stands for Integrating the Healthcare Enterprise, and is often confused with HIE, which stands for health information exchange. This can be particularly confusing, because you can use the IHE protocol to build an HIE. IHE is a second-generation HIE protocol, intended to address the limitations surrounding the man-in-the-middle architecture dictated by the HL7v2 protocol stack.

Originally, the IHE protocol, as its name suggests, was focused on the exchange of information between different types of information systems inside a single enterprise. As hospitals automated different departments, they might use one vendor to run the MRI system, another to run the laboratory, and still another to handle the x-ray machine. IHE was originally designed to get these separate systems to talk to each other.

The IHE protocol has been in development for many years and is managed by a nonprofit also called Integrating the Healthcare Enterprise. IHE is not a single protocol, but a grouping of protocols that define how different healthcare IT systems should interact. As a rule, IHE attempts not to redefine already working standards, but to specify other, already well-defined, standards where appropriate. DICOM and HL7 v3 CDA, for instance, are both leveraged in different parts of IHE. In the same spirit, some parts of the IHE standards rely on other parts. The parts of IHE are called *profiles*, so another way to say this is that "profiles extend other profiles." In order to get several vendors' health IT systems to work together, it is possible to implement each profile by software bought from a different vendor. Typically, however, a whole group of profiles (a domain or several domains) are implemented by a single piece of software.

Each IHE profile defines how a specific type of healthcare data exchange should occur. The profiles are grouped into *domains* related to medical specialties. The current domains are as follows:

- Anatomic pathology
- Cardiology
- Eye care
- IT infrastructure
- Laboratory
- Patient care coordination
- Patient care devices
- Radiation oncology
- Radiology

Each of these domains contains several profiles, which are detailed on the IHE website (*http://ihe.net*). Of these, the most important for our purposes are the ones underneath IT infrastructure (*http://www.ihe.net/Technical_Framework/index.cfm#IT*):

Audit Trail and Node Authentication (ATNA)
    Handles audit trail for HIE

Consistent Time (CT)
    Handles time sync (important for logs)

Cross-Enterprise Document Media Interchange (XDM)
   The core data migration profile; move data from point A to B using email, Direct Protocol, CD, or USB

Cross-Enterprise Document Reliable Interchange (XDR)
   Provides a standards-based specification for managing the interchange of documents that healthcare enterprises have decided to explicitly exchange using a reliable, point-to-point network

Cross-Enterprise Document Sharing (XDS)
   Contains pointers to all available records

Cross-Enterprise Sharing of Scanned Documents (XDS-SD)
   Handles scanned document sharing

Enterprise User Authentication (EUA)
   Implements single-sign on

Patient Demographics Query (PDQ)
   The central demographics store

Patient Identifier Cross Referencing (PIX)
   The master patient index (MPI) component of IHE

Patient Synchronized Application (PSA)
   User selects a patient in application A, and automatically sees the patient selected in application B, too

Personnel White Pages (PWP)
   Holds clinical "who works here" listings

Patient Identifier Cross-Reference and Patient Demographics Query for HL7v3 (PIX/ParaDQ/v3)
   Makes PIX and PDQ comply with HL7 v3 standards

Request Information for Display (RID)
   Browser-based data display

Registry Stored Query Transaction for Cross-Enterprise Document Sharing Profile
   Extends the XDS Profile with a stored query function

Retrieve Form for Data Capture (RFD)
   Handles form-based integration with research and public health

The IT infrastructure components are those components that enable complex HIE between organizations. We will discuss these components more fully. Before we leave the rest of them behind, however, take a moment to contemplate just how many different types of healthcare information systems can operate in a given enterprise. Most hospitals do not have software that performs all of these functions. Most hospitals, however, have software that performs many of these functions and rarely is all of the software from a single provider.

HIE with IHE

The IT Infrastructure profiles of IHE can work together to enable several different types of HIE, either within or between organizations. IHE is a top-down approach to HIE in the sense that software running on the network has a map of where patient records live. While IHE does require this map, it does not otherwise dictate a centralized exchange model. The map of which patient's data lives at which organization can be generated cooperatively, with each clinical organization recruiting part. The first part of HIE using IHE is using that map as a means for discovering, for any given patient, which clinical systems have relevant data. The second part of HIE involves lots of options for routing that patient data from the sending clinical information system to the receiving clinical information system.

Managing Patient Identifiers with IHE

The first component of HIE using IHE is the PIX/PDQ profiles. These two profiles are often discussed in the same breath and frequently implemented in the same software system. The patient demographics query (PDQ) is a store of patient demographic information, as understood by different parts of an HIE. The PIX is an indexing service that examines the various copies of healthcare demographics collected by the PDQ and makes determinations about which people are really the same person.

This process is at the heart of the federated health records approach to HIE. People in the United States are very concerned with the privacy implications of the federal (or any other) government having full access to their healthcare data. In many countries, especially those with socialized medicine, the Ministry of Health (or equivalent) maintains a health record, paper or electronic, for every citizen of the state. In the United States, such a centralized system, which can be very efficient when digitized properly, is unthinkable politically. As the most polar expression of American citizens' cultural distrust of government, certain far-right religious elements believe that the government handing out unique identifiers to every citizen is a step toward the destruction of the world outlined in the Book of Revelations in the Bible. The small but vocal and politically active people who believe this in the United States have ensured that no form of centralized health IT system will fly politically. Any nationally endorsed scheme for HIE must use what is called the "federated model" of managing patient identifiers.

That means that in one healthcare facility, a patient might be identified by his basic demographics and Social Security number; and in another, by a slightly different name and driver's license number. In a large HIE, a single patient might conceivably have records with slightly different demographic information and identifiers in several different clinical information systems.

When any patient visits a clinic connected to an HIE, the EHR for the clinic should query to see whether that patient has records in any other location. The PIX/PDQ component of the HIE will process this request to determine whether such patient records exist. The generalized name of this component (in non-IHE-speak) is a master patient index (MPI).

When such a query occurs, the PIX will perform an analysis of the patient demographics presented in the query against the data stored in the PDQ. The PIX will return a list of record locations that match. The PIX/PDQ does not actually have these records; they simply know which other systems in the HIE might actually possess the records.

The PIX uses algorithms to determine whether a given patient demographic search matches other records. For instance, if a PIX/PDQ is sent a search that is looking for a John Doe, who was born January 1, 1950 in Austin, Texas, then the results might have the following data:

> Memorial Medical -^-; record matches for John Doe born January 1, 1950, in Round Rock, TX
> Methodist Hospital -^-; record matches for Jonathan Doe born January 1, 1950, in Austin, TX
> Creative Clinical -^-; partial match for John Doe born January 3, 1950, in Austin, TX

Good MPI solutions are capable of recognizing that sometimes basic demographic information is recorded differently at different sites. MPI solutions understand that locations can be described differently by patients, who might say "Dallas" when they mean "Irving" or "Fort Worth" or even might say "San Antonio, Texas" when they mean "Mexico City" (which is to say, the patient might submit intentionally false information).

The purpose of the PIX/PDQ is to sort out where, on a given network, a patient might have records. A community HIE, using IHE, will set up at least one PIX/PDQ instance and use that to map the entire local HIE network.

IHE Data Exchange, the Library Model

PIX/PDQ solves the problem of what patient might be named and what systems might have records on an individual, but it is not directly involved in the core process of the exchange of records. To do that, you must actually know what clinical records are stored where, and have a mechanism for delivering those records. This process is left up to the XDS, which stands for Cross-Enterprise Document Sharing.

The analogy that is often used with XDS is the library model. XDS has two main components, the registry and the repository. If XDS were a library, the registry would be the card catalog, showing exactly what "books" (patient records) lived where. The repository would be the bookshelves themselves. In XDS, the repositories contain healthcare records that are from document sources, which in the library analogies, are like book publishers. Publishers put the books on the shelves and then update the card catalog. In IHE-speak, document sources provide records to the repository, and register the records in the registry.

It is pretty obvious how clinical users requesting documents from the HIE would pull documents from the XDS system. *Pull* in IHE-speak is to publish and discover. IHE also supports the subscribe model of HIE. NAV is a profile that provides a kind of subscription functionality to a given record in a repository. Using the technology in NAV, one provider can say, "I want to be notified of any changes to records for this patient at other hospitals." This would not be unlike a local library agreeing to give you email updates regarding books you are interested in.

IHE also has a mechanism for "interlibrary loan" called XCA (Cross-Community Access). This provides a method for members of one community network to query other IHE-based HIEs. XCA provides publish and discover functionality for exchanges outside the local area. XCA ensures that IHE is a distributed and federated health exchange protocol.

One of the most significant parts of the IHE specification, in that it overlaps with the Direct Protocol, is the XDR profile. XDR, which stands for Cross-Enterprise Document Reliable Exchange, is specifically designed to enable the exchange of documents in a push fashion, without reliance on an XDS component. This is the point-to-point component of the IHE stack. It replicates many of the features of XDS that are needed to move a set of clinical documents from point A to point B.

Both the Direct Protocol and XDR are point-to-point protocols. Of course, this could create a problem, because it potentially creates a need for two different inboxes for clinicians. Rather than support two parallel protocols functioning as point-to-point clinical message delivery mechanisms, the designers of the Direct and IHE protocols worked together to create very accurate bridging technology, so that a message could seamlessly transition from the IHE network onto the Direct network and vice versa.

These bridging methods rely on the IHE XDM, or Cross-Enterprise Document Media Interchange profile. This profile is specifically designed to support transfer of IHE messages outside of the network. The IHE to Direct bridges automatically use XDM, but XDM also supports sneaker net. Sneaker net is a humorous nickname given to the process of walking over to a computer and copying a document onto portable media and then walking it over to another computer and copying the file to the new computer. In IHE, sneaker net is supported by XDM. XDM is nothing more than a fancy compressed file that contains electronic copies of clinical documents. XDM is content-agnostic, but it will commonly contain CCR, CCD/A, or PDF files. As a result of the IHE to Direct bridges, the XDM file formats will likely be seen commonly as attachments to Direct messages.

IHE in the NWHIN

ONC has blessed IHE as one of the two officially sponsored protocols of the NWHIN. The other chosen protocol is the Direct protocol. The NWHIN will evolve into a new layer on the Internet, which we call the Health Internet. Like the original DARPAnet, the federal government is populating this new network with valuable resources. Most importantly, data from the VA, which has the largest single database of patient data in the world, will be available on the NWHIN, using the approved NWHIN protocols, IHE and Direct. The NWHIN was an effort originally started by ONC under Dr. Robert Kolodner (a card-carrying member of the VistA underground railroad). In any many ways, the NWHIN was an achievement almost as significant as meaningful use. The NWHIN contained commitments from almost every U.S. federal agency that holds significant amounts identifiable patient data, including the Social Security Administration, HHS, and the VA.

In order to facilitate this partnership, the ONC sponsored a new implementation of open source IHE software. The original project to create the reference implementation of the NWHIN IHE was called the CONNECT project (*http://www.connectopensource .org/*), and is still active. The vision of CONNECT was to implement a real-world viable interpretation of the IHE protocol stack that could be used specifically for interoperability in the United States. All of the federal agencies would join one IHE-based network and use it to communicate identifiable patient data with the other agencies.

CONNECT was a tremendous achievement, and has enabled the government agencies piloting the NWHIN to communicate patient data successfully. However, despite the CONNECT project being widely regarded as a win, the group of corporations that initially developed the codebase behind CONNECT did not win the follow-on government contract for CONNECT development. Of course, changing vendors is a reasonable thing to do on occasion, but it has significant implications for an open source project that are not issues otherwise. It is acceptable to fire a vendor, for instance, but it is not OK to freeze them out of the project development. It has become obvious that the management of the CONNECT project could not be done in an open fashion because it was subject to whims of government contracting officials who understood little about the underlying software functionality or the open source development process.

Happily, the underlying ethos of open source ensures that projects that become obviously mismanaged can take on new life through a fork. The original development community has forked CONNECT into a new project called the Aurion Project (*http://www .aurionproject.org*), which is managed by a new foundation called the Alembic Foundation (*http://www.alembicfoundation.org*). This new community is competing to attract the patronage of several of the federal agencies associated with the NWHIN, and is largely regarded as the home of the CONNECT project now. Though some federal agencies might be required to use the CONNECT project, outside organizations and HIE organizations should probably consider using Aurion, which currently appears to be the more sustainable effort.

Aurion specifically has CONNECT compatibility as a design goal, to minimize the impact of the fork. Eventually the CONNECT project, which is half open source project and half government contract, will run out of funding. Watch for interesting developments when that happens; perhaps another fork? a merger with Aurion? Who knows.

CONNECT and Aurion are not the only open source IHE efforts. The Open Health Tools (OHT) project (*http://www.openhealthtools.org/*) is home to several open source IHE components. These are professionally supported by, among others, Misys Open Source Solutions (MOSS; *http://www.misysoss.com/*). Notably, Dr. Kolodner is now the Chief Health Informatics Officer of OHT.

There are several solid implementations of IHE that exist as proprietary software. IHE is far more widely adopted as a standard in Europe, and several nations there rely on a single proprietary IHE vendor to provide HIE nationwide. This model, however, is primarily viable in nations with socialized medicine. Under that healthcare financing model it is possible to dictate the use of a single vendor nationwide. It is much easier to get instances of one vendor's IHE implementation to talk to other instances from the same vendor.

Healthcare interoperability in the United States will require connecting to multiple different vendors' IHE implementations. Given the relative immaturity of IHE as a protocol, open source implementations of IHE have a substantial advantage, as they can be more easily modified to adapt to real-world exchange problems. Moreover, the transition from the CONNECT project to the Aurion project served as strong evidence of the survivability of the open source software in this space. If you are implementing IHE in the United States, going with open source should be your default choice.

This has been a trend in health IT for several years. Though open source EHR systems are less popular than their proprietary counterparts, the need for deep customization has ensured that open source HIE options are typically more popular than proprietary options.

The Direct Project/Protocol

In a manner very similar to the CCR/CCD debate (often including many of the same players) there is a strong movement against IHE within the health IT community. Many feel that IHE is simply too complex to enable scalable health information exchange (HIE).

The alternative, which has gained substantial traction as both Microsoft and Google have endorsed it, is called the Direct Project (*http://www.directproject.org*). The Direct Project defines a simple protocol for point-to-point HIE based on SMTP protocol. Because it is based on SMTP, the Direct protocol is simple to implement using existing email-based applications. Direct is just secure email for doctors and patients. Unlike the basic assumptions of the IHE network, patients on the Direct network have all of the same privileges to make and send clinical messages that doctors do. In the Direct Project documentation this feature is often written as "patients as peers" on the network. This, as well as other technical design decisions in Direct, has made the protocol very popular with patient empowerment advocates.

Secure email has been trivial to implement for years using encryption as defined in the Secure/Multipurpose Internet Mail Extensions (S/MIME) protocol stack. However, the communication has typically been very sensitive to small changes in how S/MIME is configured. The Direct protocol enables the use of S/MIME as a health information exchange by making certain encryption configuration decisions mandatory.

Beyond mere configuration compatibility, the Direct Project implements two basic technological approaches to practically enable HIE. The first is the Direct protocol requirements for clinical attachments. Clinical documents are transferred by the Direct network just like document attachments in email. Just like attachments in email, there is no limitation to what file type can be attached to a Direct message.

This is widely regarded as one of the patient-empowering design goals of the network. If a patient wants to send her doctor a digital image, a Microsoft Word document, or a spreadsheet, the Direct network, like plain email, supports those attachment types.

However, the Direct specification also details how the network should move clinical documents in a more formal HIE. Included in these specifications is specific detail regarding how to convert to an from the IHE network. Point-to-point messaging is one of the many features of the IHE specification. IHE messages can be converted into Direct messages and vice versa. This helps to ensure that the NWHIN remains a single network, rather than having two separate messaging infrastructures. In the future, it is reasonable to expect that Direct and IHE will become even more deeply integrated.

The second major architectural innovation in Direct is the design of its trust network. The problem with HIE is that many actors in the delivery of healthcare in the United States do not actually have strong trust relationships. Sometimes this is because of ideology (i.e., Planned Parenthood vs. Catholic healthcare systems), sometimes because of competitive relationships (i.e., two hospitals in town are fierce competitors), and sometimes because of geography (i.e., California has very different rules regarding healthcare exchange than, say, Arkansas).

The Direct Project concedes that in many cases, real-world trust relationships are impossible, and does not attempt a top-down approach to trust that would try and resolve these fundamental trust differences. Instead Direct dictates that if a real-world trust relationship can be established, the Direct network can be used to securely deliver clinical messages between two organizations.

The technology that the Direct Project uses to enable this loose trust model is public key infrastructure (PKI), specifically the X.509 specifications of PKI. This is the same trust technology used to provide security between web browsers and web servers. PKI uses what are known as certificate authorities (CAs) to "vouch" for the trustability of organizations. When you use your web browser to visit your bank, your browser is asking a CA to vouch that the web server you are communicating with does in fact belong to your bank.

There is one important difference between trust enabled by the CAs in the Direct trust model and the browser trust model: there are no automatic or default trust decisions made. You can easily modify which CAs you trust in your browser, but for the most part, you decide to trust those CAs that your browser trusts by default. This means that Microsoft, the Mozilla Foundation, Apple, and other browser manufactures end up making most of the Internet trust decisions by choosing which CAs to include by default in their browsers.

In the Direct network, CAs are imported by default because no implementation would presume to make a guess about whether your organization has a clinical trust relationship with another organization. That means that Direct users have an extra burden: they must manage their own trust relationships by choosing which CAs and which other sites they trust. But this helps to ensure that no trust mistakes are ever dictated by Direct implementations.

It also means that the Direct protocol can be used internationally, or across state and national borders, with relative ease. Again, if a trust relationship can be established, communication can occur.

Practically speaking, Microsoft HealthVault is already offering Direct addresses through its PHR software to the public. In a similar fashion, Surescripts (the same people who route prescriptions) and AAFP have teamed to offer Direct addresses at large to doctors and other clinicians. More than likely, a Direct-based HIE option will be available to you before an IHE-based option is.

The PCAST Report

The President's Council of Advisers on Science and Technology (PCAST) released a report (*http://www.whitehouse.gov/sites/default/files/microsites/ostp/pcast-health-it-report.pdf*) in December 2010 that was critical of the HIE approaches that were available at the time (the Direct Project was not available when the report came out). PCAST argued that HIE should be enabled by simplified health information standards based on XML.

Generally, the health IT community regarded the PCAST recommendations as naive. Proponents of IHE-based HIE argued that PCAST was simplistic and nonstandard relative to IHE. IHE specifically accounts for the tremendous complexities of healthcare workflows in order to deliver a comprehensive solution to HIE.

Those in favor of the simplicity found in the Direct protocol found PCAST to be heavyweight like IHE, without being as well thought-out.

In short, no one in the industry could take PCAST seriously, while those outside the industry viewed the report with hope. It was widely regarded as a good effort of the top minds in "normal" IT to address the historical failings of health IT, and in many cases modified versions of the advice found in PCAST were already being implemented in either the Direct or IHE exchange efforts. However, it was immediately obvious that the PCAST workgroup, as a whole, had not done its homework on the fundamental difficulties in health IT.

The PCAST report was ultimately panned by the ONC workgroup, who was tasked to evaluate it. They decided that although the goals and ambitions found in the PCAST report were positive, there was no way for the detailed recommendations to be made compatible with meaningful use requirements in the short term.

The SMART Platform

As we mentioned in Chapter 6, many of the ideas from the Indivo X platform, which was designed from the ground up to enable peer-to-peer PHR interoperability, have been extended into an API-based interoperability scheme called the SMART platform (*http://www.smartplatform.org*).

The SMART platform provides a consistent data API in which applications can be written. This is not unlike the API that Facebook releases. Facebook's API allows applications like Farmville to access underlying social data that Facebook manages for a given user. Farmville uses that data to provide a higher level experience. In the same way, SMART enables applications to build upon a shared clinical data core.

Unlike Facebook, Google Health, or HealthVault, SMART does not make the assumption that there should be one mothership instance of the technology. Instead, each instance of the SMART platform presumes that there are other instances and that it needs to smoothly exchange clinical data between those instances.

SMART is deeply inspired by the architecture adopted in the Indivo X project and applies methods first used in the Indivo X PHR to health IT applications more generally.

Technology and Policy Were Sitting in the Tree

The automatic exchange of healthcare data using computerized processes is one of the most heated policy areas in modern healthcare informatics. HIE policy discussions are often heated and circular. Even at the highest level working groups who report to ONC, only a few people are capable technologists. Added to the problem is the fact that often, policymakers must discuss issues with health data exchange in the abstract. Instead of discussing how policy interfaces with a particular technology, policymakers must determine what rules make sense when applied to any technology. As you can imagine, this all makes for lots of circular discussions.

Unlike policy making in the abstract, we have the luxury of focusing on policy making in the context of the specific healthcare protocols. This makes the issues at least something that can be discussed in detail, rather than an entirely academic exercise. There are two important healthcare exchange network protocols that are part of the NWHIN —Direct and IHE—and they have very different approaches to how to enforce policy.

The basic policy question that must be answered for healthcare exchange to take place is "Will I send my data to this entity?" A certain high level of trust needs to be in place for this to occur. When a "sender" of health information uses the current fax system to send data, they do so assuming merely that the recipient is a trusted party under HIPAA. But with electronic health data exchange, you are not merely trusting the receiving party, you are trusting their network. Do they have adequate computer virus protection? Are they following best practices with regard to backup? Is it your responsibility to verify the status of these issues? Do you need to conduct an audit on a regular basis? Widespread health data exchange has been largely stalled in the United States because of these types of questions. For use to move forward, we need to have approaches that help ensure that providers feel safe to send data to lots and lots of other providers. They must become at least as comfortable with structured electronic health data exchange as they are currently with the fax system.

We say "at least" with a certain unease here. Frequently healthcare providers do not trust data from another provider. They feel it is important to have their lab and imaging center perform tests. Merely having the information in an XML form rather than a faxed document will not prevent the reordering of labs, if the receiving provider cannot trust the contents of the clinical document. Health IT cannot solve these problems, but it can serve to highlight and even track them. If every provider in your town, for instance, believes that a certain provider of lab results is entirely unreliable, that fact should become verifiable in the context of HIE, over time. We hope that sunlight will be the solution to many of these difficult policy questions. Both of the health information protocols provide this sunlight in different ways.

As we discussed in "The Direct Project/Protocol" on page 198, the basic approach that Direct takes to policy is the "bubble up" approach. The Direct protocol and network essentially make no automatic trust choices at all. They do, however, ensure that trust decisions are made by deciding whether or not to import x509 certificates. IHE leverages X.509 and Secure Sockets Layer (SSL) as well for its low-level connectivity decisions. That makes the X.509 certificate infrastructure the fundamental trust fabric of the NWHIN.

For both protocols, it will be the CAs that will serve to enforce policy among the holders of certificates that it issues. The federal government will have one policy to determine which CAs it decides to trust, and perhaps states or cities will either set up CAs themselves or write criteria for which CAs are appropriate. Inevitably there will be many CAs that serve to enforce many different policies on different health data exchanges between different parties.

There are efforts to create reasonable starting point policies that these CAs can adopt and enforce. The most important of these is the Data User and Reciprocal Support Agreement (DURSA). This is the legal document that formed the basis of the trial implementations of the NWHIN. Taken from the latest DURSA draft:

The Data Use and Reciprocal Support Agreement (DURSA) is a comprehensive, multi-party trust agreement that will be signed by all NHIN Health Information Exchanges (NHIEs), both public and private, wishing to participate in the Nationwide Health Information Network. The DURSA provides the legal framework governing participation in the NHIN by requiring the signatories to abide by a common set of terms and conditions. These common terms and conditions support the secure, interoperable exchange of health data between and among numerous NHIEs across the country.

Work on the DURSA has stalled somewhat, but so far, it remains a strong template for the type of document that needs to be established as a policy starting point for widespread HIE. Eventually, either DURSA, or some successor to DURSA, will need to take a remixable approach to health IT policy that was first extensively tested with the Creative Commons content licenses. The Creative Commons licenses allow artists, writers, photographers, and other content creators to license access to their copyrighted works in one of several different ways. There are several variants of the Creative Commons licenses that serve content creators with different philosophies in different situations. But because the licenses are standardized, content consumers can make only a few decisions about what licenses they are comfortable with. The alternative is to have every content creator license their copyright differently, ensuring that content consumers will never be able to safely consume content en masse.

Eventually, DURSA must evolve into something similar. There are only a few reasonable decision points that will work for HIE policy in different circumstances and for broad interchange to occur, parties must be able to evaluate only a few different common policy options to determine what they are comfortable accepting.

When a party decides to trust a CA, say the CA for the state of Texas, they are saying that the policies enforced by that CA are policies they are comfortable accepting, and that they are comfortable with the level of policy enforcement that the CA practices. As a result, especially for Direct, which requires little setup beyond certificate import, the decision to import a certificate from a CA is equivalent to a whole set of policy decisions that amount to, "Yes, we can exchange identifiable patient data." This is the link between health IT policy and technology. Given that politics, and not technology, has kept health IT back for the last three decades, if there are issues that could derail the NWHIN/Health Internet, and the widespread exchange of health data, this is the area where those problems would occur.

CHAPTER 12

HIPAA: The Far-Reaching Healthcare Regulation

Doctors and administrators evaluating health IT software frequently ask, "Is it HIPAA compliant?" We usually answer, "You tell us what it means to be HIPAA compliant, and we will tell whether or not the software is." HIPAA is probably the most ironic acronym in healthcare. It stands for the Health Insurance Portability and Accountability Act. Although HIPAA has succeeded largely in making health information more "accountable," it is usually the first excuse for not making it portable.

The regulation of health IT systems has long been a complex and evolving area. Ultimately, the courts and the choices by regulators about what to really enforce determine what any regulation really means. Recent court cases and enforcement have created a much more solid context for defining just what regulations mean. Previously, the federal government was criticized for lacking enforcement for HIPAA and other health-IT-related law. HITECH—the same law that created the meaningful use funding—has changed this, providing new mechanisms for enforcement that should ensure that regulations will really stick. This chapter looks at HIPAA, with a nod to some other federal laws. Each state has a collection of laws that can be just as important to know for your state.

The first basic task is to gain an understanding of how health IT is affected by HIPAA. There at least two reliable ways to do this. The easy way is to read the summaries that HHS provides for the HIPAA security and privacy rules (*http://www.hhs.gov/ocr/pri vacy/hipaa/understanding/index.html*). They lay out most of what you need to understand. For those who prefer the hard way, you can gain an even deeper understanding by reading the actual regulations yourself. This way, you do not take our word, or that of anyone else, regarding what the regulations actually say.

So far, the regulation is short enough that a technically informed layman can skim through it pretty quickly. Most of the law applies to processes and training that have nothing to do with health IT. Print it out and then use a highlighter to mark sections that you do not understand, or that you feel are especially important in your environment. As you do this, remember that we said reading HIPAA was useful and possible for a layman, but we did not say it would be fun.

Review these resources with your own environment in mind and make notes as you go over the content. At the end of this exercise, you might feel that you have everything well in hand or, alternatively, that you really need a healthcare lawyer. A specialist lawyer will understand HIPAA as a living document, subject to interpretation by judges and juries, but you should do some work to be prepared for that level of insight. You will be better off hearing a health lawyer's advice with your own understanding of the law. Consider first asking your lawyer to explain what you did not understand about the literal text, so that you can have some confidence in your own understanding. Many in the healthcare world choose not to hire expensive lawyers and opt instead for seminars and other less expensive ways to ensure compliance. Either way, too much discussion of HIPAA is based on what the regulation ought to say, rather than what it does say. Reading the regulations, or at least the HHS site, can help you.

Regulators and the courts understand that the technology is moving faster than the regulations can keep up. If you are operating in a fashion that is in keeping with the spirit of the regulations, which are generally designed to enforce respect for patient privacy, then you will probably be fine. This is not a blank check by any stretch of the imagination, but if you are doing something innovative, can demonstrate you are trying to protect privacy as best you can, and are not obviously violating the law, you probably do not have anything to be worried about. (This is just an observation, of course, not legal advice.)

On the other hand, if you are ignoring your responsibility to read the rules, and you are not following industry best practices or the laws in question, keep in mind that these regulations come with serious fines and in some cases potential jail time. This is something to take very seriously, as the HITECH act has made the already stiff penalties of HIPAA far more potentially painful. Make no mistake: if you flout HIPAA, it could land you in prison or bankrupt your organization. Take it seriously.

With that in mind, we begin our discussion of health IT regulations with HIPAA, the most significant and expansive health privacy law in the United States.

HIPAA is a bundle of provisions that touch on numerous health industry matters, passed by the U.S. Congress during the Clinton administration in 1996. Although the law created substantial changes in the healthcare industry, it has lain somewhat dormant until recent years. Only recently has HHS begun seriously enforcing the rule, a laxness that has postponed the court decisions that normally end up determining what the details of any law actually mean in practice. Moreover, the HITECH act also modified the provisions of HIPAA substantially. Hopefully this will allow us to discuss the law in a way that will not be quickly outdated. Still, the law changes quickly, and it is important to use recent resources when creating a compliance plan.

Does HIPAA Cover Me?

The first thing to understand about HIPAA is that it does not cover all healthcare data or all people who know something about a patient's health.

HIPAA was put in place to protect the privacy of individuals from the enormous power that players in the healthcare industry have, relative to other people in our lives. If you tell Aunt Jenny that you have a serious healthcare condition, Aunt Jenny can walk right into the offices of a major newspaper and hire out an ad that details your health problem for the world to see. You might call telling your Aunt Jenny a secret a "privacy choice," specifically a "bad privacy choice." HIPAA has nothing to say about that. Your doctor often knows information about your health before you do, and often knows information that you would prefer that no one knows, but that you must share to get healthcare. As a natural result, your doctor has a tremendous amount of data without you having made any kind of privacy choice. HIPAA places a burden on your clinical providers, and other "covered entities" in the healthcare system—health insurance companies and health care insurance claims clearinghouses—to restore a patient's ability to make privacy choices.

Generally, HIPAA covers anyone who is obviously in a position of power regarding your health data, but does not cover Aunt Jenny or anyone else with whom you might consider sharing your secrets. HIPAA comes into play when a healthcare provider or other covered entity has been given, or generates, healthcare data about a patient. Then, and only then, does that entity have certain obligations regarding that data under HIPAA.

Moreover, HIPAA extends to organizations and persons with whom that entity shares that data, organizations and persons known as business associates. So most of the discussion regarding any given data point should begin with, "Is this data HIPAA-covered?" Happily, this question is rarely hard to answer. If you are providing IT services to the healthcare provider as an employee, all data the patient gives you and all data you generate about the patient is always covered. If you are not an employee (and often even if you are), you will be asked to sign what is known as a Business Associate Agreement, which will spell out clearly that all data you receive from the covered entity is HIPAA-covered. HITECH has several provisions that put those given secondary access to patient data (business associates in HIPAA speak) on a largely equal footing with the original HIPAA covered entity. If you come in contact with patient data that is HIPAA covered, you are a HIPAA covered entity of one kind or another, and must have appropriate policies and procedures in place to handle this patient information appropriately.

For most readers, that can serve as the end of the discussion on when HIPAA does and does not apply.

If the preceding discussion does not sufficiently clarify your position, you can use a general rule of thumb: if you are involved with the generation, routing, or processing of electronic medical billing, you are probably a covered entity under HIPAA. That includes clearinghouses and medical billing companies that route medical bills, payers that receive medical bills, and of course healthcare providers who originate the electronic bills. If, somehow, you are still not sure given this rule of thumb, then you need to carefully read the document that provides complete flowcharts answering this question (*https://www.cms.gov/HIPAAGenInfo/Downloads/CoveredEntitycharts.pdf*).

If you are still not sure, act as if you are covered (by putting a hold on any sharing of patient data) until you can consult with a lawyer who specializes in healthcare law.

If at this point, you are sure that your health information service is not covered by HIPAA—congratulations, your life will probably be much easier. You are probably providing a PHR, or legally speaking, you should consider yourself one. From a legal perspective, a PHR is software that stores patient health information obtained either directly from the patient, or from another organization following a request from that patient to release that information. Ironically, the patient's right to request and receive this data is also detailed in another part of HIPAA. You are basically in the same boat with Aunt Jenny: you get health data as the result of a patient choosing to give you that data. Contract law, user agreements, or a privacy policy covers your obligation to patient privacy.

Even if you are a PHR, you still need to care about HIPAA! The HITECH act created new rules, enforced by the Federal Trade Commission (FTC; HIPAA is typically enforced by HHS) regarding breach notices. The FTC breach notices will be discussed shortly. We'll see more reasons as we go along.

Responsibilities of Covered Entities

At this point, you should feel comfortable knowing that you either are or are not a HIPAA-covered entity. The industry term for data that is protected under HIPAA is protected health information (PHI). As a covered entity, you have PHI, and you need to take steps to protect it. HHS often refers to e-PHI to delineate PHI on computers. Note that PHI is either identifiable or easily reidentifiable. If you truly separate the identity of the patient from a set of health data, that health data is no longer PHI. Truly separating PHI from the identity of the patient is called deidentification and is much harder than it seems, and you should assume that you have not done so successfully until you are absolutely certain that you have.

The HIPAA regulations list 18 categories of identifying information; if a record has even one of them, it cannot be considered deidentified. They range from the obvious (patient name, date of birth, Social Security number) to the less obvious (IP address, state of residence, age if the patient is over 90), to the typical government catch-all (anything else that could be used to identify a patient).

HIPAA allows deidentified data to be shared freely, primarily to enable research. If you are guessing about whether you have truly deidentified a set of patient data, you are playing a very dangerous game. Here is a rule of thumb for deidentification: If you are using an algorithm to deidentify patient data, it had better be more reliable than a human doing the same process.

HIPAA came with two titles. Title I is all about changes to regulation for health insurance, and will not be covered here. The second title directed HHS to create several "administrative simplification rules" that would improve the handling of healthcare data. Out of this process came at least five rules covering the following:

- Privacy
- Transactions and code sets
- Security
- Unique identifiers
- Enforcement

Of these, we can dismiss some as not relevant to our discussion on health IT. The enforcement rule, for instance, details how enforcement will take place, and sets penalties for infractions of other rules. For our purposes it is enough to say that HIPAA is enforced and that penalties can be very stiff, including jail time for blatant offenders (*http://www.ama-assn.org/amednews/2010/06/07/bisb0607.htm*).

The transactions and code sets rule dictates specific code sets for electronic billing. These are discussed in Chapter 3 and Chapter 10.

The unique identifiers rule creates a unique numbering system, called the National Provider Identifier (NPI) system, for all healthcare providers and healthcare plans in the country. Every doctor or other healthcare provider who either prescribes medications or bills Medicare, Medicaid, or other health insurance is required to have an NPI. As a result, almost all healthcare providers have NPI records. Moreover, many of the corporations involved in the delivery of healthcare are listed in the directory. The NPI directory is published, including updates, each month from the National Plan and Provider Enumeration System (NPPES) website (*https://nppes.cms.hhs.gov/*). The NPI directory is also available as a RESTful API resource (*http://docnpi.com*), which is more fully discussed in Chapter 10.

The privacy rule has few direct health IT implications, but forms the heart of HIPAA's aspirations with regard to privacy. Moreover, new requirements created by meaningful use essentially require automation of what previously were manual operations under the HIPAA privacy rule.

The bulk of specific health IT regulation takes place in the security rule. This is where the law specifies things like encryption standards. Computer security professionals should be well-versed in the language of the security rule, the contents of which are readily understandable by those with IT training. For healthcare professionals, the requirements of the security rule can be somewhat intimidating, because it uses very specific terminology regarding information security in many of its requirements.

The HHS summarizes the responsibilities detailed in the security rule for covered entities like this:

- Ensure the confidentiality, integrity, and availability of all e-PHI they create, receive, maintain, or transmit.
- Identify and protect against reasonably anticipated threats to the security or integrity of the information.
- Protect against reasonably anticipated, impermissible uses or disclosures.
- Ensure compliance by their workforce.

That is a perfect 10,000 foot summary.

A more detailed examination of the security and privacy rules, along with amendments to HIPAA from the HITECH act, the current and future requirements of meaningful use, and a healthy dose of industry best practices, allows us to create the following list of requirements for health IT systems. Because we are mixing what you are legally required to do with industry standards and common sense here, you cannot use this discussion to calculate your legal responsibilities, but this does make for a pretty good starting to-do list. It takes you above and beyond HIPAA compliance, and although it might be legal to ignore parts of this advice, you should have a very good reason for doing so, and probably have hired a lawyer to make certain that what you were ignoring was prudent.

- The core goals are confidentiality, integrity, and availability (CIA) for PHI. Learn the meaning of CIA in relation to patient data, embrace its implications, and recognize that in health IT we are responsible for best practices and not just legal compliance. Doing the minimum here will eventually burn you. A good rule of thumb is that it's usually spending money in the long run to achieve better security —so long as you spend it on things that really matter, and not just a false sense of security. If better security comes at the costs of patient care, you have some fudge room. If you are obviously embracing security costs that do not impact patient care (i.e., a properly maintained firewall and antivirus software), regulators and enforcing agencies might be more lenient when you make choices to ignore security best practices in a way that obviously benefits patients.
- Patients have the right to get copies of their health data within 30 days of a request. Meaningful use requires mechanisms for patients to receive this data in both electronic and paper form. EHR and other health IT systems should probably support several modes of export, including sending data to a tethered PHR (defined in Chapter 6), emailing the patient record to the patient on the Direct network (see Chapter 10), providing an electronic copy on a burned CD-ROM or USB stick, and printing the contents of the electronic record clearly. One of the most substantial fines ($4.3 million) ever levied for HIPAA violations concerned this simple issue (*http://www.hhs.gov/ocr/privacy/hipaa/enforcement/examples/cignetpenaltynotice .pdf*).

- Patients have the right to make amendments to the contents of their health records, if they view the data as incorrect or incomplete. Eventually, meaningful use will likely require that this occur using HIE mechanisms. Mechanisms should be in place to note that certain data has "patient comments" or that certain data is "patient sourced." Data that comes directly from a patient controller PHR should never be excluded from the core record even if it is viewed as inaccurate (as opposed to other data coming in from the HIE). Most important, even modifications to paper charts should have electronic logs, so that you can demonstrate compliance with the "patient amendment" rule.

- Patients have the right to get a list of all the disclosures of their health data. A disclosure here means that a covered entity shares HIPAA-covered PHI with another organization. When a doctor sends clinical information to a health insurer for payment, for instance, that counts as a disclosure under HIPAA. HITECH extends this to include detailed reporting of electronic data disclosures over the last three years. It is a good bet that this disclosure will someday need to be delivered in an electronic format. (e.g., Direct, CD-ROM, USB). One ethical procedure that goes beyond compliance with this rule is to simply include the patient in all communication regarding the patient. There is no reason that all electronic communication regarding the patient could not be copied and automatically sent to the patient, too. This becomes much simpler as the result of the Direct Project. (However, I am *not* suggesting you copy the patient on all communication or disclosure —think about how many minute disclosures and shares there are in the course of an episode of illness. See the author's call for restraint (*http://www.jopm.org/opinion/commentary/2011/07/05/sharks-bees-and-health-privacy-paranoia/*) on interpreting privacy rules. Notification for disclosures, no matter what approach is taken, can never be completely automated. Some HIPAA disclosures, related to warrants for instance, must not be reported to the patient.

- Covered entities must appoint a privacy officer and have a mechanism to receive complaints regarding HIPAA violations or requests from patients who want to exercise their rights under HIPAA. It is reasonable to assume that regulations will eventually require digital accounting of the work performed by this individual.

- There must be a privacy policy in place, overseen by the privacy officer, and audited annually by this officer for compliance.

- There must be a security policy in place, with yearly audits to enforce compliance. These audits should specifically perform risk analysis, which evaluates the risks to e-PHI against the technologies used to protect that e-PHI in an ongoing basis.

- Both the security and privacy policies and their audits should specifically cover e-PHI.

- Those policies that are sitting on the shelf collecting dust in the boss's office do not cut it. HITECH has substantially changed HIPAA, and those who do not update their policies and procedures to match may be regarded as "willful neglectors."

- You should have HIPAA audits whenever you have a HIPAA event and at least yearly otherwise. Keep the results of the audits, and the changes you make as the result of your audits, for at least six years.

- Your policies should include how to respond to issues discovered during audits.

- Both the security policies and the privacy policies should encompass the process of hiring and firing employees. There should be some digital log that shows that when an employee left an organization, his access to clinical information systems containing PHI was removed.

- Classes of employees must have access to classes of PHI. In the IT security industry this is called role-based access control. If everyone has access to all clinical information, you must specifically justify why this was needed in some kind of dated and formal document. Your billing and scheduling staff, for instance, do not need full access to the patient record to do their jobs. They need access only to the data needed to perform their jobs, and both policy and software should enforce these limits. HHS calls this level of access "minimum necessary." Attempts to circumvent these boundaries should be logged. HHS calls this "access controls."

- Regularly train staff regarding the handling of PHI, including e-PHI.

- If your organization hands over PHI to a business associate, you must have some policy to ensure that basic protection is being taken with regard to the PHI you have provided.

- You have obligations to protect the accessibility and integrity of the PHI under your care. You must have an emergency plan to ensure that PHI is not lost in case of an emergency. Remember that an emergency can mean anything from a hurricane, to an act of war, to a simple hard drive failure. Your plan for recovering PHI should include off-site encrypted backup. Because encryption makes backing up more unstable, your emergency plan should include at least yearly "test restores" to verify that off-site encrypted backups can be re-created without access to anything on-site. (For instance, if you keep your encryption keys on-site and you lose that information when you are hit by a tornado, it does not help you to have off-site encrypted backups). HHS calls this "integrity controls."

- You must limit access to physical copies of health data (both paper files and EHR servers, etc.). You should probably have systems in place for logging physical access to healthcare data, although this might be prohibitively expensive. At a minimum it should require traditional, metal keys to access servers storing e-PHI.

- You should generally have a physical access plan that includes facility security plans and logs of visitor sign-ins and escorts. Of course, you really need to escort guests, assuming they would otherwise be able to access information systems containing PHI. For simplicity, your patient workflow should never allow patients to wander into areas that contain servers with PHI. No guest access control or logging system will be effective if strangers can physically access an area containing PHI media.

- Electronic access to PHI should be limited and logged. Given the importance of the uptime of clinical systems, this logging should be part of a comprehensive logging and monitoring strategy. If someone asks you whether Dr. Smith accessed John Doe's electronic patient record last Tuesday, you should be able to definitively answer that question. HHS refers to this as "audit controls."

- Because you are required to log certain events to be HIPAA compliant, it might be possible that PHI is slipping into the logs themselves. It is not, in itself, PHI for your log to read: "Dr. Smith accessed patient record #111111 last Tuesday." But if it reads "Dr. Smith accessed the record for John Doe last Tuesday," or if the log ties patient record #111111 to John Doe elsewhere, the log is PHI, and must be kept private. And if your system logs *might* contain PHI, they must always be treated as though they *do* contain it. The very fact that a person is attending your clinical facility is technically PHI, and that means if you have the name of a person other than a staff member in your logs, it should be presumed to be PHI unless proven otherwise by an internal audit. For simplicity, try to keep patient names and birthdays out of the logs.

- You need a strategy to ensure that patients and guests will not be able to see other patients' health information on screens. Usually that means screen savers with passwords, and monitors that cannot easily be viewed by patients and guests. It also means that there should be some type of auto-logout mechanism in your EHR. Be aware of what "pops up" on screens when people log back in. Again, even the fact that a person is a patient is generally considered PHI. If a patient sees a neighbor's name on the screen after a clinician dismisses the screen saver, that is considered a breach. This issue becomes more important as clinicians consider using computers to go over the electronic record with the patient in the exam room. This is a wonderful idea, but you must ensure that no patient names continue to be visible when the next patient enters the room.

- When being transferred across open networks, PHI must be encrypted. The Internet, obviously, is an open network. If you fail to have a properly configured firewall, or if you have a rogue WiFi hotspot, your network might be classified as an open network. (This is especially true if it becomes obvious that you knew you had a leaky firewall or rogue hotspot.) Most agree that network traffic should be encrypted where possible, even across local networks, to protect against a "closed" network suddenly becoming an "open" network. HHS calls this "transmission security."

- You must have mechanisms in place to protect against data erasure, both accidental and purposeful. Your backup strategy is an important part of this, but if data can be deleted at the EHR level, and this deletion is then replicated to backups across lower-level backing systems, you might have a problem.

- Engage in ongoing risk management. Suppose you decide that you are going to use Mac OS X on your network to avoid getting an antivirus solution. If viruses targeting Mac OS X become common, your risk management process should pick up on that fact and you should invest in OS X antivirus technology. The environment changes, and your IT processes should change, too.

- When you are retiring hardware of any kind, assume that it has PHI on it and erase all data completely. You do not want to be that guy who sold a populated EHR server on eBay accidentally, and yes, it has happened. Have a policy that specifically mandates that decommissioned servers, workstations, laptops, cell phones, and portable drives are all erased before being retired. For most organizations, especially smaller ones, it is simpler and less expensive to assume that every computer or device has PHI than to track which ones have PHI. If something can store digital information, and it is being thrown away, wipe it just in case.

- Although HIPAA "trumps" less restrictive state-level privacy laws, HIPAA and other federal and state privacy laws sometimes conflict. The general rule is that whichever rule is more protective of patient privacy prevails. It is not always easy to identify which one that is, however, and you do not want to get caught in a turf war between federal and state regulators. If you find that your reading of state law and HIPAA collide, hire a health care IT lawyer. This type of issue is precisely what their expertise is for. HITECH provisions allow state attorneys general to enforce HIPAA, and to provide funds to state governments through HIPAA-related fines.

- HIE is wonderful, but different states have very different laws regarding how to handle PHI. Merely transferring certain health data across state lines could get you in legal hot water. In some cases, even different cities within different states have different rules.

- Computer viruses have a unique ability to negatively impact the integrity of PHI. An ad-hoc, consumer-grade antivirus strategy might work for smaller sites. If you have more than 50 computers in your clinical organization, you probably need to have some kind of centralized antivirus solution. If you have more than 100 computers, lacking centralized antivirus software would probably be regarded as irresponsible.

- If a device is mobile, or might be, encrypt it if you can. Prefer whole-drive encryption approaches, because this ends up being simpler for end users. Do not presume to know which mobile devices will be used for PHI and which will not. There are too many good, cheap encryption technologies (e.g., TrueCrypt; see *http://www .truecrypt.org/*) to neglect this. If a mobile device cannot easily support encryption, make sure that your training emphasizes that such mobile devices should never store PHI. Alternatively, you can ban mobile devices entirely: no laptops, smartphones, or USB sticks allowed. This type of approach is unlikely to be well-received or easy to enforce, though.

- Recognize that encryption is not a data-loss prevention strategy. It is a data-loss *mitigation* strategy. There is evidence to suggest that data encryption does not actually reduce the incidence of data loss (*http://weis2010.econinfosec.org/papers/ses sion1/weis2010_tucker.pdf*)). Many organizations underinvest in important efforts to protect patient data because they are "encrypting it." But remember that if you lose the encryption keys along with the encrypted data, the encryption does not help much. If you are encrypting data on your central EHR server, and you encrypt the network connection to your workstations, you still need to worry about copy and paste. Most of the time, privacy breaches are based on either clear human error, or in some cases, insiders who are intentionally betraying the trust the institution has placed in them. Either way, the encryption cannot protect your patients' privacy if the people who have the "keys" are either intentionally or unintentionally failing to protect the data. If you have to choose between good training and background checks or encryption, focus on the human element, and postpone the deployment of encryption.

- When using encryption to protect health data, default to encryption built the on NIST-approved AES 256-bit standard. This standard, also called Rijndael by the Belgian developers who invented it, seems to have won the widespread admiration of several different HITECH-related standards. However, specific encryption standards can become dangerous to rely on overnight. Pay attention to news announcing a new standard from NIST replacing AES 256, but for now it is the gold standard.

HIPAA: A Reasonable Regulation

Many of the requirements mentioned here, and specifically in HIPAA, are "addressable" rather than required. That means that you have to follow the recommendation, provide a reasonable alternative, or document why you did nothing. Generally, if you have to do something that the law forbids because of some extenuating circumstance, document the event carefully as an exception to policy and do not try to hide it from auditors. If you are required to report events, do so in a timely manner. Doing otherwise could mean that you are guilty of "willful neglect," which mandates that HHS deliver a stiff penalty if they find out. Screw up and be honest, and you will suffer some. Screw up and hide it, and you will suffer greatly.

The specific wording on the distinction between "addressable" and "required" from the HHS website is worth repeating:

> Covered entities are required to comply with every Security Rule "Standard." However, the Security Rule categorizes certain implementation specifications within those standards as "addressable," while others are "required." The "required" implementation specifications must be implemented. The "addressable" designation does not mean that an implementation specification is optional. However, it permits covered entities to determine whether the addressable implementation specification is reasonable and appropriate for that covered entity. If it is not, the Security Rule allows the covered entity to adopt an alternative measure that achieves the purpose of the standard, if the alternative measure is reasonable and appropriate.

Moreover, it is worth detailing exactly what HHS has to say regarding the vastly differing resources that different clinical environments can offer.

HHS recognizes that covered entities range from the smallest provider to the largest, multi-state health plan. Therefore the Security Rule is flexible and scalable to allow covered entities to analyze their own needs and implement solutions appropriate for their specific environments. What is appropriate for a particular covered entity will depend on the nature of the covered entity's business, as well as the covered entity's size and resources.

HHS intends HIPAA to be interpreted and implemented differently at different sites. No one should think that a "one-size-fits-all approach" will work with HIPAA compliance. In reality, there are hundreds of different approaches to HIPAA compliance that would probably pass muster with an HHS audit, and there are hundreds of approaches that would seem right but that they might find wanting.

Given that HHS is being reasonable regarding your resource constraints, it becomes worthwhile to approach HIPAA compliance with some ingenuity.

Duct-Tape HIPAA Strategies

Just because you are following regulations does not mean that you have to be stodgy or traditional or lay out a lot of money. Veterans Affairs, after some very embarrassing incidents where patient data was lost because of stolen laptops, has created one of the most draconian information security schemes on the planet. This has had a twofold effect. First it is nearly impossible to get anything unusual done in the VA environment. USB sticks do not work, web browsers are stuck at ancient versions, and so on. Ironically, because it is nearly impossible to get anything done, many who work at the VA tend to work around the rules, by working outside the VA network.

Being draconian about security ensures that your users will revert to silent rebellion. If it becomes apparent, in a legal situation, that management was aware of this kind of policy-reality dissonance, the benefits of a super-strict policy can quickly be negated. Instead try to find solutions to difficult problems by thinking outside the box. A common policy at the VA and other institutions with strict polices is to forbid normal USB sticks. USB sticks are really useful for countless tasks that have nothing to do with PHI, so forbidding them only marginally improves security (they normally do not have PHI anyway) and dramatically reduces productivity.

Instead of forbidding the use of USB sticks, make their use safer. Use the following methods to ensure that when a USB stick containing PHI is lost, you can be certain that its contents were encrypted, and it is much more likely that the USB stick will be discovered.

First train your staff on how to use TrueCrypt, or some other encryption product of your choice, to safely store PHI on USB drives. Then visit the hardware store and buy several large chunks of sanded plywood (larger than 15 inches by 15 inches, so that it would be very difficult to fit in a backpack or briefcase). Using a permanent marker, write the following on both sides of the plywood: "This USB key is to be used internally at Acme Clinic only. Please do not take me home. Please always encrypt me with True-

Crypt/Whatever. If found outside Acme Clinic, please return to Acme Clinic at 1000 Acme Way, Houston, TX. 77004 (713)111-1111 for a $100 no-questions-asked reward."

Drill a hole in the corner of each plywood piece and use a large key ring to attach the USB key to the large key ring. Make sure both the USB key ring and the USB key are very sturdy. Put a QR code sticker on the USB key itself with the same "reward if found" content embedded. Also put a plain-text file called *readme.txt* on the drive with the same information.

The problem with USB sticks and laptops is that well-meaning employees accidentally take them home and then get their backpacks or briefcases stolen. By having a very inconvenient keychain and a constant reminder to use encryption with the USB stick at all times, you can get all the benefits of an in-clinic sneaker net, without the problems associated with wanton USB stick use. Make it clear that regular USB sticks are strictly forbidden, and back that up with audits of USB mounting logs. Name the USB keys something like XYZAcmeClinicUSB1 so that when they are mounted on a computer they can be differentiated from outside USB sticks.

You can easily make 10 of these using sturdy USB drives bought in bulk for under $100. This, plus the use of TrueCrypt on all Windows laptops and servers and the whole-disk encryption technology that is built into most modern Linux servers, makes a viable alternative to an enterprise encryption architecture that could cost hundreds of thousands of dollars.

Consider marking your in-house laptops with similarly garrulous markings. (For heaven's sake, do not mark a laptop as potentially having PHI without also encrypting the laptop's hard drive.)

HIPAA does not require you to encrypt your servers. However, mass deployment of encryption across every computer in your environment can sometimes be easier than just encrypting laptops. Having a policy that enforces the use of inexpensive, open source hard drive encryption technology can be a much cheaper alternative to purchasing an encryption management system that can effectively manage an environment where some systems are encrypted and other systems are not.

Almost all networking security components such as firewalls, network intrusion detection systems, and antivirus products have robust open source alternatives that can save an organization tremendous amounts of money, assuming they are competently maintained. Alternatively, Microsoft provides slightly more expensive products that almost always work together well and might need less maintenance. In either case, any clinical organization is going to need help merging the traditional work of IT (just keeping computers running) and health IT (keeping EHRs and their satellite systems running). Make sure that your "normal" IT people are working in concert with your health IT people. An HHS HIPAA audit is a bad time to learn that your organization's technical people were conducting a turf war at the expense of properly handling PHI.

Consider bringing in an outside team of lawyers and health IT consultants to do a mock audit to identify holes in your system that you are too close to see.

Breach Notification Rules

If you have a breach of HIPAA-covered patient data, you must report it, both to HHS and to the patients whose data was breached. Moreover, the FTC enforces the same rules for non-HIPAA-covered PHR providers. The breach notification rules are one of the most significant new regulations on the PHR industry.

There are several magic numbers to remember regarding breach notification: 500, 60, and 10.

If a breach of unsecured PHI occurs that impacts more than 500 patients, a covered entity or PHR provider is required to report the breach more quickly, within 60 days, and is also required to notify the media. Large breaches are essentially automatically made public information on the HHS online "wall of shame." Remember, a single lost laptop or USB device could easily contain information for thousands of patients. This is the reason that the industry is so concerned with device encryption. PHI on an encrypted device is not considered unsecured and therefore no embarrassing notification is necessary in the event a device is lost or stolen—it's not considered a breach.

If fewer than 500 unsecured records are breached, you can save some embarrassment. In this case you only need to report the breach to HHS or the FTC and, of course, the patients involved in the breach.

This brings us to the magic number 10. If, when attempting to contact patients for whom breaches have occurred, it is discovered that contact information for more than 10 of the patients is out of date, then the breach must also be published either in a major newspaper where the patient lives, or on the home page of the clinical provider. Of course, this could be even more embarrassing than the notices required when more than 500 records are lost.

As a result of this rule, PHR companies especially have been much more careful to gather alternative means of contacting consumers. Breach notices can be sent to patients via first-class mail or email, assuming the patient has agreed to electronic notices. As a result of the breach notification rules, many clinics and hospitals in the United States have begun asking for email addresses for patients for the first time. PHR companies frequently require two email addresses as well as a postal mail address for patients as a result of the new rules.

The FTC definition of a PHR company broadly includes the notion of anyone offering to manage health information for consumers on the Internet. Specifically, from an FTC site on the Health Breach Notification Rule (*http://business.ftc.gov/privacy-and-secu rity/health-privacy*):

If you have an online service that allows consumers to store and organize medical information from many sources in one online location, you're a vendor of personal health records.

This rule likely applies to anyone setting up shop as a PHR, a patient social network, or any other service that "manages health information" for consumers. It is unclear, at this point, just how broadly the health and fitness industry will be covered under the rule.

If you are a health information service provider who is supporting a PHR or a HIPAA-covered entity, then no matter how many people were involved, you have only 60 days to notify that entity and allow them to initiate their own disclosure responsibilities. For most part, as a PHR or covered entity, if your business associate has a breach, your responsibilities are the same as if you had a breach. As a business associate or service provider, mere notification to that entity is not sufficient; you must confirm that the entity actually got the message.

In Summary

For the seasoned security professional, HIPAA can seem like a lightweight regulation.

For the most part, HIPAA simply mandates some very high-level requirements regarding your policies, your workflows, and the audits that ensure that the two are continually connected. The goal that your policies and audits should seek is to keep the outsiders entirely away from PHI, without interfering too much with the work that the insiders need to do with that PHI.

CHAPTER 13

Open Source Systems

Open source software is not currently found in many healthcare settings in the United States, although the infrastructures of healthcare systems in several other countries run on it, and one of the most celebrated EHRs in the United States—the Department of Veterans Affairs' VistA—is open source. The role of open source is expanding quickly, and providers are soon going to find themselves using open source software for many everyday functions—perhaps without realizing it, because it might be buried inside proprietary offerings.

The meaning of open source software, also often called *free software*, is often misunderstood. These systems distribute all the resources needed to continue developing and using them to the public. If the original developer should vanish, or insist on taking the software on a path that some of the users dislike, any user can hire programmers to continue development. The key characteristic of open source systems is *not* that they are cost-free. Although their source code is available without charge, practical deployment often requires considerable investment, and most users choose to contract with businesses that charge for deployment or maintenance. The key characteristic of open source is that it responds to the needs of the users instead of the vendors, and successful open source systems develop communities that control its future.

Why do we devote a whole chapter to open source, given that it is currently barely a blip on the healthcare radar? The authors have to admit to some personal interest here: we have both spent our healthcare careers building and promoting open source systems. But more fundamentally, open source is poised to become a major part of the healthcare field, and it is critical for readers to see that coming. The CONNECT and Direct projects, sponsored by the ONC at HHS, ensure that the crucial process of document exchange will become an open source area. Other projects, including some described later in this chapter, also show promise.

Why Open Source?

We state categorically that healthcare benefits from open source more than any other industry. Our claim rests on the first and major observation we make in this book: the diversity of healthcare organizations. Some encompass a single doctor in a rural setting; others are enormous conglomerates. Some offer expensive, specialized treatments to tiny populations and others rush through thousands of people with no ability to pay every day. Each specialty is totally different in its practices, terminology, and interaction with patients. Patients move between family practitioners, hospitals, rehab centers, nursing homes, and other diverse organizations. Pediatricians deal with babies (and their families) while gerontologists deal with the elderly (and their families). Different states and countries have different payment systems, diagnoses, demographic profiles, and privacy policies.

In short, healthcare requires, more than any other field, tremendously flexible and extendable systems—which is what open source thrives on.

Proprietary vendors need to standardize. They provide a lowest common denominator to customers. Although small, new vendors try to react quickly to customer requests; the vendors get more bureaucratic and less interested in the needs of the individual customer as they grow. With open source software, each user can make the changes it needs. Up-front investment in programmer time might be greater with open source software, but the software ends up exactly as the user wants. In addition, the advances created by one user are freely shared with all others, amortizing costs. Furthermore, unlike most staff, programmers can be hired from far away, so a national and even global market exists in software customization. (That said, you usually need a programmer on site to interact intimately with staff if you want the software to fit your workflow perfectly.)

The authors' experience in healthcare provides one overarching generalization about healthcare organizations and IT: they are extremely ignorant and conservative with IT decision making, an aloofness that costs them dearly. Counterintuitively, healthcare is one of the most innovative and experimental industries when it comes to tools and techniques for patient care. But in health IT systems, one consistent and very successful (for the IT vendor) business model stands out: lock-in.

A vendor creates a system so specific, nonstandardized, and esoteric that one and only one vendor can possibly support or maintain it. The vendor then pursues aggressive sales strategies, often combined with low initial pricing. Once fully established in the customer site, the vendor can drain the customer with ever-increasing maintenance and upgrade fees. Any decision by the facility to change systems is severely limited by the exorbitant integration fees, export fees, and lack of cooperation by the existing vendor to migrate data to another system.

What is truly shocking is healthcare's decades-long adherence to this business model, which has experienced relatively limited windows of success in other industries. The authors can count hundreds of instances where facilities chose to break free from one vendor's lock-in model, only to walk into arms of another with the same model.

The authors sincerely hope that this book can encourage people with strong IT backgrounds to enter healthcare and apply long-known and hard-earned lessons on purchasing and implementing complex systems to an industry in desperate need of it. Meaningful use presents the perfect opportunity for fresh air, as it applies a basic level of standardization and has received generally positive feedback from the industry as a whole.

For the open source tools to thrive and develop useful features, it is crucial that they receive feedback and participation from a variety of stakeholders. It can be intimidating to present pilot projects to administrative bodies within a healthcare agency, but without internal champions and a willingness by those bodies to accept some level or risk, we will waste the potential for a viable open source ecosystem in healthcare. As we stated in the introduction to this book, it is difficult to think of another industry that literally required incentives (bribes) from the federal government to adopt electronic systems, which most other industries have chosen to adopt for competitive advantage or are clamoring to adopt.

Open source has proven to be a systematic and comprehensive model for innovative, sustainable, and explosive growth. The Web itself, and all of the leading companies in today's technology sector, including Google, Apple, and Facebook, are built directly on various flavors of open source underpinnings, such as Linux, MySQL, Apache, and a range of new technologies, sometimes developed by those famous companies and released to the public under open source licenses.

More than 10 years ago, when ClearHealth was fighting for its first customer, the idea of open source in large reputable organizations was still very much an uncertain concept. But 10 years in this age of technology is a millennium in terms of progress. Healthcare must adopt a more modern and cyclical view of IT if it is to survive in any recognizable form for another 10 years. Everyone in the industry can see that current costs, expenditures, and relationships across all layers are headed to bankruptcy at a frightening pace. IT alone is not a savior, but the meaningful use goal of an efficient, accurate, and innovation-seeking methodology presents a destination that can control healthcare costs while substantially improving patient care.

Major Open Source Healthcare Projects

The rest of this chapter explores the most important open source projects that the authors currently find in health care. We look briefly at each one's history, its status in relation to standards, and how to obtain it. This information is constantly changing and is accurate at the time of writing, but will almost certainly change and expand after this book is published.

When evaluating IT systems, many organizations attempt to look at the credibility of the organization behind it. That is a completely reasonable measure, but is often confused with adept marketing by those organizations. ClearHealth has been owned and operated for 10 years by the same organization without changing hands. One notable proprietary system has been similarly owned for 10 years or more, eClinicalWorks. The cannot be said of Centricity by GE, NextGen, or AllScripts, all of which have changed hands and business models, some more than a half-dozen times in the past 10 years.

To date, only three systems with an open source license have received certification for meaningful use.

ClearHealth

ClearHealth (*http://www.clear-health.com*) started out as a response to David's background in enterprise resource planning systems and other complex deployments, which led him to seek opportunities for similar innovation in the healthcare market. After exploring several of the open source systems present at the time and contributing significantly to a few (including OpenEMR, which still exists), he saw a clear need for a system built with current and extendable infrastructure that could scale to an enterprise level.

ClearHealth was created in a collaboration with Operation Samahan in San Diego, California, which still runs it today. That shows the power and long-term sustainability created by open source systems. Any look at the long-term costs of a facility like Operation Samahan shows the irrefutable advantages of open source.

ClearHealth offers the Advantage 3.1.5 version system, which was certified for meaningful use compliance in December 2010 by InfoGuard, a CMS-recognized Authorized Testing and Certification Body (ATCB). It is certified for comprehensive use in outpatient facilities and is the only system needed for meaningful use compliance. The Advantage system includes a comprehensive practice management suite as well as a comprehensive EHR suite. It also offers tailored modules for general practice, OB/GYN, dermatology, oncology, physical therapy, behavioral health, public health, and a few other select lines of care.

The Advantage system version 3 is based on the VistA system originally created by the VA and covered in more detail elsewhere in this text. It is a web-based system that supports all major version web browsers.

For inpatient facilities, ClearHealth also offers the WebVista system, which will receive certification for meaningful use in December 2011.

The open source repository of ClearHealth source code is available from Github (*http://www.github.com/clearhealth*). Forums for open source users are on the ClearHealth website (*http://www.clear-health.com/forum*).

Mirth Connect

Mirth Connect (*http://www.mirthcorp.com/products/mirth-connect*) is a "Swiss Army knife" healthcare integration engine that serves as a glue between various IT systems employed by healthcare facilities. Transitioning from legacy systems to more flexible ones, in particular, can be challenging and time consuming, and during that process of transition Mirth Connect is an invaluable tool to help integrate data between systems. In many scenarios, data can be received or transmitted to partners who are outside the control of the facility and might be using improperly configured, out-of-date, or non-standards-compliant systems. Primarily supporting the HL7 communication standard, Mirth Connect provides an infrastructure to translate to and from those systems with comprehensive support for most of the standards that make up meaningful use guidelines.

Mirth Connect is open source under the Mozilla Public License 1.1. The corporation's website offers both an open source repository of Mirth Connect code (*http://www.mirthproject.org/svn/*) and user forums (*http://www.mirthcorp.com/community/forums/*).

VistA Variants and Other Certified Open Source EHR Systems

Most hospital-grade open source EHR projects are based on VistA, although we will also mention several that are not. Several of the important VistA-based projects have achieved meaningful use certification.

ClearHealth (*http://www.clear-health.com/*) has derived some components directly from VistA and has slowly been rewriting VistA in the PHP programming language. ClearHealth was the first product to achieve comprehensive certification and is certified for outpatient use. See*http://onc-chpl.force.com/ehrcert/EHRProductDetail?id=a0X300000025W61EAE*.

DSS (*http://dssinc.com*) is a government contractor (primarily working on VistA for the VA) that has turned into an open source EHR vendor with VxVistA (*https://www.vxvista.org/*), which is certified for inpatient use. See*http://onc-chpl.force.com/ehrcert/EHRProductDetail?id=a0X30000003l3dlEAA*.

Medsphere (*http://www.medsphere.org*) is an open source VistA vendor supporting the OpenVistA stack, and its OpenVistA Carevue product is certified for inpatient use. See *http://onc-chpl.force.com/ehrcert/EHRProductDetail?id=a0X30000003kEUmEAM*.

WorldVistA (*http://www.worldvista.org*) is a nonprofit that has achieved certification with both the inpatient and outpatient versions of its WorldVistA EHR. See *http://onc-chpl.force.com/ehrcert/EHRProductDetail?id=a0X30000003ld0lEAA* and *http://onc-chpl.force.com/ehrcert/EHRProductDetail?id=a0X30000003lNCPEA2*.

Interestingly, one of the oldest VistA forks was not done by a company, but by another federal agency. Indian Health Services (IHS) forked VistA to create its Resource and

Patient Management System (RPMS; see*http://www.ihs.gov/RPMS/*). Because some IHS clinics qualify to received meaningful use subsidies, IHS has applied for and received full certification. Several other private organizations outside IHS are using RPMS, which is also available under FOIA, to achieve meaningful use. See*http://onc-chpl.force.com/ ehrcert/EHRProductDetail?id=a0X30000003jg3XEAQ*.

Several other open source projects, including OpenEMR (*http://oemr.org*) and Tolven (*http://www.tolven.org*), are currently partially certified and plan to achieve comprehensive certification.

PopHealth (*http://projectpophealth.org/*) is a Ruby on Rails project from the MITRE Corporation, and probably the only project with the intent of targeting only partial certification. PopHealth is not intended to be used as an EHR, but rather to support all of the clinical quality measure reporting that is required by meaningful use, using exports from standard CCR or HITSPC32 records of EHR patient data. See*http://onc -chpl.force.com/ehrcert/EHRProductDetail?id=a0X30000003lxJlEAI*.

This list of open source projects that have achieved meaningful use certification is unlikely to be comprehensive. We are not including proprietary versions of VistA that have been certified, as well as versions of OpenEMR that have been certified but are offered only as ASP services. Most important, the tool for searching for certified systems, available at *http://onc-chpl.force.com/ehrcert/CHPLHome*, does not support searching by open source status. It is likely that other open source projects we have not heard of appear on this list.

There is no reason to imply that open source EHR systems are of better quality than the hundreds of certified proprietary EHR products, but the open source ones do publish their source code. This means, for instance, that if the original vendor fails to achieve an upcoming stage of meaningful use certification, customers can hire programmers to do the job themselves. If you are a developer and you would like to see what type of systems are required to achieve certification, these applications are a good place to start. All of the systems included here either have a freely downloadable version that is equivalent to the certified version, or intend to soon. In some cases, the software vendors will choose to certify only their commercial open source offerings.

OpenMRS

While this book has almost exclusively focused on systems that thrive in the United States, there is one Open Source EHR project that has the opposite focus that deserves mention: OpenMRS.

OpenMRS (*http://www.openmrs.org*) is probably the most important EHR outside the United States. It a well-architected Java-based EHR solution specifically designed to meet the needs of low-resource clinical environments. While it is capable enough to be used in large hospital-like environments, it is also designed to work in a clinic that is nothing more than a tent, with a tacklebox full of medications. In the United States, its development is backed by the Regenstrief Institute, Partners in Health and the Rockefeller Foundation. It has received endorsements and code contributions from organizations as large as UNICEF. However, while these names certainly sound impressive and speak to the intellectual pedigree of the project, what is amazing about OpenMRS are not its backers but rather its implementers. The project's codebase is almost entirely engineered by geeks who are on the ground in the various countries where it is deployed. OpenMRS has a simple technology rule. If a technology choice does not support its "grown locally" development model, another option is chosen. It has been successfully installed in hundreds of clinics all over the world.

Ironically, it can be argued that the OpenMRS EHR model is one of the best available in any Open Source solution, precisely because the project has no interest in being deployed within the United States (although this has not stopped several U.S. installations). While OpenMRS is utterly unconcerned with the Meaningful Use standards in the US, it is also has no interest in billing subsystems, CPT codes, ICD codes, or any of the other health IT anchors imposed by the United States healthcare system. As a result, the OpenMRS project is free to pursue whatever technological/clinical design actually works on the ground. In a moment of project Zen, OpenMRS has achieved real meaningful use precisely by ignoring the meaningful use standards. Its impact on the health IT space outside the United States can hardly be understated.

Meaningful Use Implementation Assessment

The assessment in this appendix estimates the level of difficulty your organization will have in adopting and complying with the meaningful use guidelines. The form is intended to be completed by an organizational administrator for the entire hospital or clinic. An individual assessment form will appear elsewhere in this book. Please make your best guess for your site or department as a whole.

Staff Skills Assessment	No Experience	Some Experience	Average Experience	Expert
Experience with electronic prescriptions				
Experience with electronic clinical notes				
Experience with clinical rules systems				
Experience with coding using CPT procedure codes				
Experience with coding using ICD9 diagnostic codes				
General computer competence				
Experience with electronic signing				
Organizational workflow assessment	None of the time	Some of the time	Most of the time	Always
Consistent vitals signs collections				

Collect detailed demographics				
Perform electronic clinical reporting				
Conduct internal HIPAA and security audits				
Provide patient education materials				
Perform medication reconciliation				
Provide patients receipts with coding				
Most patients for the same condition are treated consistently regardless of provider				
Claims are transmitted in-house by staff electronically				
Interoperability	Not available	—	—	Available
Order labs electronically		—	—	
Electronic lab results		—	—	
Send electronic data such as PDF, CCR, or CCD		—	—	
Receive ElectronicData such as PDF, CCR, or CCD		—	—	
Report immunizations electronically		—	—	
Information technology	False	—	—	True
Organization has 1 or more full-time IT staff members		—	—	
IT staff has experience with heterogeneous systems (Windows, Mac, Linux)		—	—	
Organization owns and operates servers equipment without intermediaries or consultants	False	—	—	True

Desktop equipment is up to date, refreshed every 3-5 years		—	—	
Your organization has successfully completed a large health IT implementation before		—	—	
Tally your score				
	Total items in this column above	Total items in this column above	Total items in this column above	Total items in this column above
Subtotal				
	Carry total below	Multiply subtotal above by 2	Multiply subtotal above by 3	Multiple subtotal above by 4
Total Score				

Consult the following categories to see our estimate about how ready your organization is to proceed with meaningful use adoption.

Total Score 30 or Below

Unfortunately, the odds are not good that your organization can complete a direct implementation of meaningful use compliance and be successful without first addressing some fundamental areas of organizational readiness. Low-hanging fruit that will improve your readiness commonly include basic staff training for computer proficiency, modernization of equipment, and hiring or reorganizing your IT staff to have tighter integration into your organization. To avoid this, put the IT foundations in place before investing in a meaningful use project.

Be warned that, in general, large IT implementations fail 50% of the time. You should expect that even if you embark on a project and it is successful, you will require 8 to 16 months to be compliant.

Total Score 31-60

There are some significant considerations you should take into account before embarking on meaningful use adoption. You might want to consider spending 6 to 12 months improving some of the fundamental aspects of your organization. Our experience shows that preparatory projects, such as interoperability, increasing staff proficiency, and improving in-house IT, are better addressed as general organizational initiatives than by sweeping them into a meaningful use implementation. If you try to do them all at the same time as meaningful use, they become big distractions from the EHR and workflow concerns at the heart of meaningful use.

You should expect to be 6 to 12 months from the start of your project before you are compliant. Meaningful use projects in organizations with this IT maturity are likely succeed only about 60% of the time.

Total Score 61-90

For the most part, your organization is well equipped to embark on a project to become meaningful use compliant. But do not underestimate the amount of organizational energy, cost, and time it will take to reach that point.

You should expect 4 to 10 months from the start of your project before you are compliant.

Total Score 91 and above

Although never an easy process, adopting meaningful use guidelines and reaching compliance for your organization probably involves only changes to existing processes you currently operate, rather than entirely new systems and wholesale changes to workflow. It is still a good idea to be meticulous and thoughtful in the planning of your implementation, and not to be overly optimistic about how quickly it can be done or when you can benefit from incentive payments.

You should expect 3 to 6 months from the start of your project before you are compliant.

 Be cautious of vendor promises about the time it will take, and especially wary of any deals or discounts that are really loans against future meaningful use incentive payments. In our experience, those types of deals have left organizations with overly expensive implementations and inattentive vendor relationships.

About the Authors

Fred Trotter is a recognized expert in free and open source medical software and security systems. He has spoken on those subjects at the SCALE DOHCS conference, OSCON, LinuxWorld, and DefCon, and is the MC for the Open Source Health Conference. He has been quoted in multiple articles on health information technology in several print and online journals, including Wired, ZSnet, Government Health IT, Modern Healthcare, Linux Journal, Free Software Magazine, NPR and LinuxMedNews. Trotter has a B.S. in computer science, a B.A in psychology, and a B.A in philosophy from Trinity University. Trotter minored in business administration, cognitive science, and management information systems. Before working directly on health software, Trotter passed the CISSP certification and consulted for VeriSign on HIPAA security for major hospitals and health institutions. Trotter was originally trained on information security at the Air Force Information Warfare Center.

David Uhlman is CEO of ClearHealth, Inc., which created and supports ClearHealth, the first and only open source, meaningful use-certified, comprehensive, ambulatory EHR. Coming from a background of supply-chain systems and big business ERP for companies including DEC, Micro Systems, Motorola, and EDS, David entered healthcare in 2001 as CTO for the OpenEHR project. One of the first companies to try commercializing open source healthcare systems, OpenEHR met face first with the difficult realities of bringing proven mainstream technologies into the complicated and sometimes nonsensical world of healthcare. In 2003 David became CEO of ClearHealth and created the ClearHealth system based on VistA that was originally developed by the Veterans Health Administration.

ClearHealth's software is open source (GPL) and powers more than 1,000 sites from small offices to mega-institutions servicing millions of patients per year. As CEO of ClearHealth Inc. David also oversees outsourced management and operations consulting of several general practice groups and in 2013 will begin operating it's own general practice facilities.

A frequent speaker and writer David has presented and OSCON, TEPR, LinuxWorld, SCALE, OSHC, and others. You can see his work online in Modern Health Care, Wired, Linux Journal, and on his blog: Health 365.

Get even more for your money.

Join the O'Reilly Community, and register the O'Reilly books you own. It's free, and you'll get:

- $4.99 ebook upgrade offer
- 40% upgrade offer on O'Reilly print books
- Membership discounts on books and events
- Free lifetime updates to ebooks and videos
- Multiple ebook formats, DRM FREE
- Participation in the O'Reilly community
- Newsletters
- Account management
- 100% Satisfaction Guarantee

Signing up is easy:

1. Go to: oreilly.com/go/register
2. Create an O'Reilly login.
3. Provide your address.
4. Register your books.

Note: English-language books only

To order books online:
oreilly.com/store

For questions about products or an order:
orders@oreilly.com

To sign up to get topic-specific email announcements and/or news about upcoming books, conferences, special offers, and new technologies:
elists@oreilly.com

For technical questions about book content:
booktech@oreilly.com

To submit new book proposals to our editors:
proposals@oreilly.com

O'Reilly books are available in multiple DRM-free ebook formats. For more information:
oreilly.com/ebooks

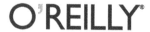

O'REILLY®

Spreading the knowledge of innovators | oreilly.com

Have it your way.

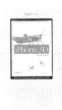 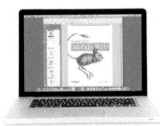 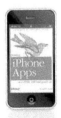 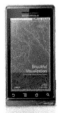
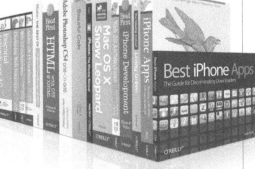